Time-Varying Effect Modeling for the Behavioral, Social, and Health Sciences

Stephanie T. Lanza
Ashley N. Linden-Carmichael

Time-Varying Effect Modeling for the Behavioral, Social, and Health Sciences

Springer

Stephanie T. Lanza
Edna Bennett Pierce Prevention
Research Center
The Pennsylvania State University
University Park, PA, USA

Ashley N. Linden-Carmichael
Edna Bennett Pierce Prevention
Research Center
The Pennsylvania State University
University Park, PA, USA

ISBN 978-3-030-70943-3 ISBN 978-3-030-70944-0 (eBook)
https://doi.org/10.1007/978-3-030-70944-0

This Springer imprint is published by the registered company Springer Nature Switzerland AG
The registered company address is: Gewerbestrasse 11, 6330 Cham, Switzerland

For Sadie and Maura,
who inspire me every day.

STL

For Brad,
who has offered time-invariant love and support.

ANLC

Acknowledgments

We are incredibly grateful for the support of our many colleagues. We would first like to thank Drs. Runze Li and John Dziak for their key intellectual contributions to time-varying effect modeling, including the development and documentation of the %TVEM SAS macros. We are also grateful to Dr. Gregory Fosco for sharing his FLOW daily diary dataset for use in Chapter 6 and to Dr. Mengya Xia for her assistance in analyzing these data. We greatly appreciate our colleagues' helpful, critical, and encouraging reviews of our chapters along the way, most notably Natalia Van Doren, Dr. Melissa Lippold, and Dr. Scott Graupensberger. We are grateful for the support and brainstorming of our Addiction and Innovative Methods lab team members—including Anna Hochgraf, Samuel Stull, and Dr. Renee Cloutier. We would also like to thank Amanda Applegate for her meticulous edits and colorful figure-making. Lastly, we would be remiss if we did not acknowledge the constant encouragement of our colleagues in the College of Health and Human Development and at The Pennsylvania State University more generally; we are grateful to have had such a supportive work environment in which to write this book.

Contents

Chapter 1
A Conceptual Introduction to Time-Varying Effect Modeling

This book is the first to introduce applied researchers to an extension of multiple linear regression, time-varying effect modeling (TVEM). TVEM can be used to advance research on developmental and dynamic processes by examining how associations between variables change across time. The primary goal of this volume is to introduce readers to new research questions that can be addressed by applying TVEM to their own research. Our hope is that readers will gain the practical skills to specify a wide variety of time-varying effect models, including those with continuous, binary, or count outcomes, as well as those using cross-sectional data, repeated cross-sectional data, panel data, or intensive longitudinal data (ILD). Throughout the book, emphasis is placed on interpreting the output provided by TVEM.

We present numerous original empirical examples based on data from studies with different designs and include outcome variables with different distributions. We also direct the reader to published papers to see additional examples that resemble studies they may wish to conduct. This volume is an ideal resource for researchers interested in addressing new questions about time-varying effects. It is appropriate for graduate students in the social, behavioral, developmental, and public health sciences who have, at a minimum, completed a graduate-level statistics course on regression analysis.

The companion website for this book (https://prevention.psu.edu/books/tvem/) contains a variety of resources, including links to a SAS macro for conducting TVEM and its corresponding users' guide. Syntax used to generate all-new empirical analyses presented in this book is provided on the website so that researchers may copy and modify it for use in their own work. We also provide a recommended reading list with links to the articles where available.

S. T. Lanza, A. N. Linden-Carmichael, *Time-Varying Effect Modeling for the Behavioral, Social, and Health Sciences*,
https://doi.org/10.1007/978-3-030-70944-0_1

1.1 What is Time-Varying Effect Modeling?

TVEM is a statistical method that researchers can use to answer a number of new, important research questions about how the relationship between two variables changes over time. TVEM has been applied to research questions in the social, behavioral, and health sciences and has been gaining popularity for its ability to provide more refined answers to research questions that address how the associations between constructs differ flexibly across time. Time-varying regression coefficients can be estimated such that the nature of change over time can be complex and nonlinear, and need not be specified a priori. Because of this complexity, figures are used to graphically summarize the value of a coefficient over continuous time. By identifying points in time (e.g., ages) at which individuals are at increased risk for adverse outcomes and points in time at which risk factors are most strongly associated with those outcomes, TVEM can inform optimal timing for targeted intervention.

Most fundamentally, questions to be addressed using TVEM must have "time" in mind, or else a more traditional analysis such as linear regression may be sufficient to address one's research questions. Let us begin with a thought exercise. Suppose one launches a short-term marketing campaign for a retail chain in certain stores and wishes to track the differences in daily store revenue on days leading up to, during, and after the campaign. In this scenario, mean differences in daily revenue across stores with and without the campaign could be modeled using TVEM. The effect of the campaign on revenue likely would not be expected to have a sudden, steady impact, but rather to increase in the days following the campaign, with a period of significant effect and eventual dissipation of that effect. The flexibility of coefficient functions estimated across time in TVEM lends itself to revealing the time-varying effect of the marketing campaign on revenue as it naturally strengthens and weakens across days. Further, this approach provides confidence intervals, enabling significance testing across continuous time. Store characteristics, such as the average income of households in the surrounding neighborhood or years of experience of the store manager, could be included to determine whether the time-varying effects of the campaign differ according to these characteristics. Perhaps stores in more affluent neighborhoods experience, on average, a greater impact on revenue as a function of the campaign compared to less affluent neighborhoods, but only during the first few days. This type of nuanced investigation about factors that may be associated with an outcome across time is exactly the type of question TVEM was designed to answer.

The concept of time, and its operationalization, is central to TVEM and must have an inherent meaning (i.e., time must be on a ratio scale, represented by a real number with a meaningful zero point). In the example above, one may wish to estimate the effect of the marketing campaign on daily revenue across days during and after the launch of the campaign. The effect likely would be expected to change across days, yet the shape of that expected change might be difficult to specify a priori. Rather than estimating, say, linear change in the effect across days, TVEM can reveal any natural ebbs and flows in the effectiveness of the marketing campaign. Thus, defining a zero point for different types of time is critical in TVEM. In other words, a crucial first step in specifying and testing a time-varying effect model is centering the time variable or defining a meaningful zero point on the time scale.

Throughout this book we refer to *real-time* (i.e., clock/calendar time, typically relevant for studies with an intensive longitudinal design); *developmental time* (i.e., age); *historical time* (data drawn from different times across history, such as annual Monitoring the Future (MTF; Johnston, O'Malley, Bachman, Schulenberg, & Miech, 2014; Miech et al., 2020) data from 1976–2020)); and *time relative to an event* (e.g., time since intervention, time relative to becoming a parent). The zero point for time in a developmental study, where age is the time metric, often is defined at the *time of birth* (age 0). In this case, time scores would be positive numbers across all individuals and assessments unless one re-centered time so that age 0 corresponded to a different age of participants during the study (e.g., age 30). Alternatively, a zero point in a developmental study might be defined more contextually, such as timing of high school graduation (graduation timing coded as time = 0). In such a model, the interpretation would be made in terms of *time relative to an event*. A variable is created to indicate the number of seconds, hours, years, etc., prior to or since the event, and 0 indicates the event time (in this case, timing of graduation). If an intervention was administered, then 0 typically would be coded to reflect the timing of that intervention start or completion, keeping in mind that assessments completed prior to the intervention can be coded using negative numbers indicating time until the event. If examining historical time and the year of data collection is the time variable, then 0 truly means *year 0* (i.e., more than 2000 years ago!). However, we suggest that re-centering the years so that 0 falls within or near the years being studied thus benefitting both computation and interpretation. If one is analyzing ILD (e.g., many assessments within day), time could be defined as *real-time* (e.g., clock time, time of day), in which case 0 might correspond to 12:00 AM, with all values of time coded as the number of hours or minutes that have elapsed since midnight. However, more meaningful zero points might exist, such as time since waking, time since taking medication, or time since last cigarette.

In some studies, ILD is collected either to gain more reliable estimates of an association between variables or to examine the variability from moment-to-moment in that association. In such studies, it may not be appropriate to align the data by centering time at the study start time and then estimate a time-varying association. This would only make sense if one wishes to test a hypothesis about systematic changes in an association across time in study. If the assessments were designed to capture random samples of time throughout and/or across days, one may not expect there to be a systematic trend in the coefficients across time in study. However, if the assessments span a period of time in which an event of interest occurs, it may be useful to center time such that Day 0 corresponds to the day of the first observed event. We present such an example in Chap. 6.

1.1.1 *Time-Invariant Covariates vs. Time-Varying Covariates*

Naturally, the outcome (or dependent variable) in TVEM is assumed to vary with time, however time is defined for that study. Covariates (or independent variables) included in TVEM however may be either time-invariant or time-varying. Some covariates, like sex or treatment condition in a randomized controlled trial, tend to be stable over time and often are measured only once. Others, like the level of craving experienced during a smoking quit attempt, can change quite quickly or dramatically over time. To capture variability on such covariates, they need to be measured repeatedly in a longitudinal or intensive longitudinal study.

Covariates are variables of scientific interest because they may have an impact on the outcome of interest. These can be things that are constant or changing. If we study the process of quitting smoking, craving is a covariate because it is associated with the outcome. Craving is a time-varying covariate because the intensity can vary almost constantly. Other variables, like sex, racial/ethnic group, and socioeconomic status, may impact how much someone smokes while trying to quit, but are typically considered time-invariant covariates.

1.1.2 *Time-Invariant Effects vs. Time-Varying Effects*

The association between a covariate and the outcome may change over time. Time-varying effects of time-varying covariates typically are considered in TVEM. Although it may seem counterintuitive, a variable that does not vary over time also can have effects that do vary over time. This is perhaps the easiest to think about when we consider intervention effects. In a randomized controlled trial, a person typically is assigned either to a control group or an intervention group, and their assignment does not change. But the difference between the control and intervention groups in an outcome—or the treatment effect—can vary over time. This variation is a time-varying effect. Consider a youth program designed to have a lasting impact on reducing behavior problems at school. In this example, the treatment may be more effective early in the trial (i.e., producing a larger effect on behavior problems) but become less effective as time goes on. Again, the *effect* of a covariate can vary, regardless of whether the covariate is time-varying or time-invariant. Table 1.1 presents hypothetical research questions that correspond to each type of covariate and effect; all are expressed in the context of modeling daily data on the level of craving smoking during a quit attempt across 3 weeks of data.

Table 1.1 Hypothetical questions that can be addressed with regression, multilevel modeling, or TVEM depending on the type of covariate and type of effect specified

		Type of effect	
		Time-invariant	Time-varying
Type of covariate	Time-invariant (e.g., sex)	Do female and male participants generally have different mean craving on the last study day? *TVEM not indicated; can be addressed with regression*	Do male and female participants differ in their mean craving at any point throughout the 3-week period? If so, when? *Can be addressed with TVEM*
	Time-varying (e.g., activity level)	Do individuals generally have different mean craving levels on days with higher activity level? *TVEM not indicated; can be addressed with multilevel modeling*	What is the pattern of the association between daily activity level and daily craving across the 3-week period? *Can be addressed with TVEM*

1.2 TVEM as a Simple Extension of Linear Regression

To explain the mathematical model in TVEM, we start by walking through a simple example that builds upon linear regression. Linear regression is perhaps the most commonly used statistical analytic technique researchers use to address quantitative questions. Suppose one is interested in examining career satisfaction in adulthood and has access to a large, cross-sectional dataset of adults across ages 18–65 that includes a valid and reliable score of career satisfaction. In a very simple time-varying effect model, one might specify an intercept-only regression model to estimate the mean level of career satisfaction (SAT_i, where i indexes the individual), as follows:

$$SAT_i = \beta_0 + \epsilon_i$$

The interpretation of the intercept coefficient, β_0, is the estimated mean career satisfaction in the population, and the error term, ϵ_i, reflects individual i's deviation from that mean. To examine the association between covariates and career satisfaction, we can add any number of covariates to this model to estimate linear associations among variables. For example, to examine sex differences in mean career satisfaction we can add a dummy variable for sex (SEX_i, coded 1 = male, 0 = female for each individual i) as a covariate in the above model:

$$SAT_i = \beta_0 + \beta_1 SEX_i + \epsilon_i$$

Now the intercept, β_0, is interpreted as the mean career satisfaction associated with being female, and the coefficient for sex, β_1, represents the estimated difference in mean career satisfaction associated with being male. It then follows that our estimated mean career satisfaction for male adults equals $\beta_0 + \beta_1$. In this model, the error term, ϵ_i, reflects individual *i*'s deviation from their sex-specific mean. This model assumes that the errors are independent across individuals.

Suppose that a dataset includes each individual's age (say, to the nearest whole number, AGE_i). The equation above makes another key assumption that is often not given careful consideration: that the estimated association between sex and career satisfaction, β_1, is the same across all ages. In other words, the model implicitly assumes that the sex difference in mean career satisfaction is equally applicable in young adulthood (e.g., age 18), older adulthood (e.g., age 65), and every age between. Suppose one wanted to test a psychological theory that predicts an increasing sex difference in career satisfaction throughout adolescence and young adulthood, but the theory lacked specificity in terms of the ages at which that gap increased. One possibility is to add a main effect for age and an interaction term for the product of age and sex, as follows:

$$SAT_i = \beta_0 + \beta_1 SEX_i + \beta_2 AGE_i + \beta_3 SEX_i * AGE_i + \epsilon_i$$

This indeed allows for such a test of the theory, but we would be making another important assumption—that the male–female difference changes in a constant, linear manner across age. Such an assumption of linear change over time (in this case, age) in the strength of an association has limited what we know about many studied associations, as it may obscure more complex trends over time. An alternative approach would be to use TVEM to estimate the coefficient for sex as a nonparametric (i.e., not linear, quadratic, or other parametric form) function of age. The following TVEM equation shows the elegant and conceptually simple extension to the linear model:

$$SAT_i = \beta_0(t) + \beta_1(t) SEX_i + \epsilon_i$$

Here, the intercept and the coefficient for sex are both specified to vary flexibly with age, as indicated by the *t* added after each coefficient to indicate time. Essentially, this model estimates the coefficient for sex as a function of ages 18–65, making only an assumption that there are no discontinuities in the coefficient function (we will discuss ways to explore prespecified discontinuities or break-points in coefficient functions, in Chap. 2). So rather than the results providing a single-number summary, or point estimate, for the intercept and another for the coefficient of sex (i.e., for the association between sex and career satisfaction), TVEM provides a nonparametric coefficient *function*, or flexibly changing curve, for the intercept (in this case, mean career satisfaction for female adults across age) and another coefficient function for the association between sex and career satisfaction across age. These coefficient functions are summarized graphically by plotting their values and corresponding 95% confidence bands over continuous time.

Note that we indicated that age was to the nearest year, yet the coefficient functions are estimated as a function of continuous time or age in this case. Data need not be truly continuous across time; TVEM uses all available information from which to estimate a smooth curve across time. The more densely the time (age) range is sampled, the more accurate the estimate at that time point along the smoothed curve. And thus, for time points at which fewer data points are available, the confidence intervals will tend to be wider.

As with traditional multiple linear regression, TVEM can accommodate complex features, such as multiple covariates, interaction terms, repeated measures, sample weights, and link functions to predict binary and count outcomes. These features will be discussed in later chapters.

1.3 Empirical Example: Age-Varying Associations Between Sexual Minority Status and Suicidal Behavior Across Ages 18–60

To demonstrate the concepts of TVEM more concretely, next we describe the research questions and summarize selected findings from a study by Fish, Rice, Lanza, and Russell (2019) that appeared in a special issue of the *Prevention Science* devoted to the developmental period of young adulthood. In this study, suicide-related behaviors were modeled as a function of sexual minority status, with the effect of sexual minority status specified as age-varying. The overall goals of this study were to examine suicide-related disparities between sexual minority adults and heterosexual adults in the US (i.e., the estimated association between sexual minority status and suicide-related behaviors), identify critical ages at which disparities are greatest, and examine individual characteristics that may moderate the association between sexual minority status and suicide-related behaviors across age. In addition, the study examined, among sexual minority adults only, the link between sexual identity and suicide-related behaviors. This information could provide improved targeting of suicide preventive interventions based on age.

The authors used cross-sectional data from the National Epidemiologic Survey of Alcohol and Related Conditions-III (NESARC-III; Grant et al., 2014), a nationally representative sample of US adults, to examine age-varying group differences in suicidal behavior across ages 18–60. Sample weights were used so that findings would be more representative of the population of adults. Such a large sample size (weighted $n = 27{,}768.6$) is not typically necessary for TVEM, but this study attempted to examine how the intersection of suicidal behavior and sexual minority status varies across ages spanning more than four decades. Approximately 10% of the population was categorized as sexual minority using an inclusive approach based on responses to items about same-sex attraction, same-sex behavior, and identifying as lesbian, gay, or bisexual (LGB). Thus, an overall sample of this size provided a unique opportunity to reliably unpack the potentially complex association between suicidal behavior and sexual minority status in the general population. Further, sex (i.e., male, female) was examined as a moderator of the age-varying association between sexual minority status (the independent variable) and suicidal behavior (the dependent variable). If we think of the difference in suicidal behavior between heterosexual individuals and sexual minority individuals as a health disparity, we can think of the age-varying association between sexual minority status and suicidal behavior as an age-varying health disparity. The moderation analysis, then, can be thought of as identifying individual characteristics that are associated with this age-varying health disparity.

Figure 1 of the results reported in this original published study (Fish et al., 2019), reproduced here as Fig. 1.1, shows the estimated percent of adults reporting suicidal

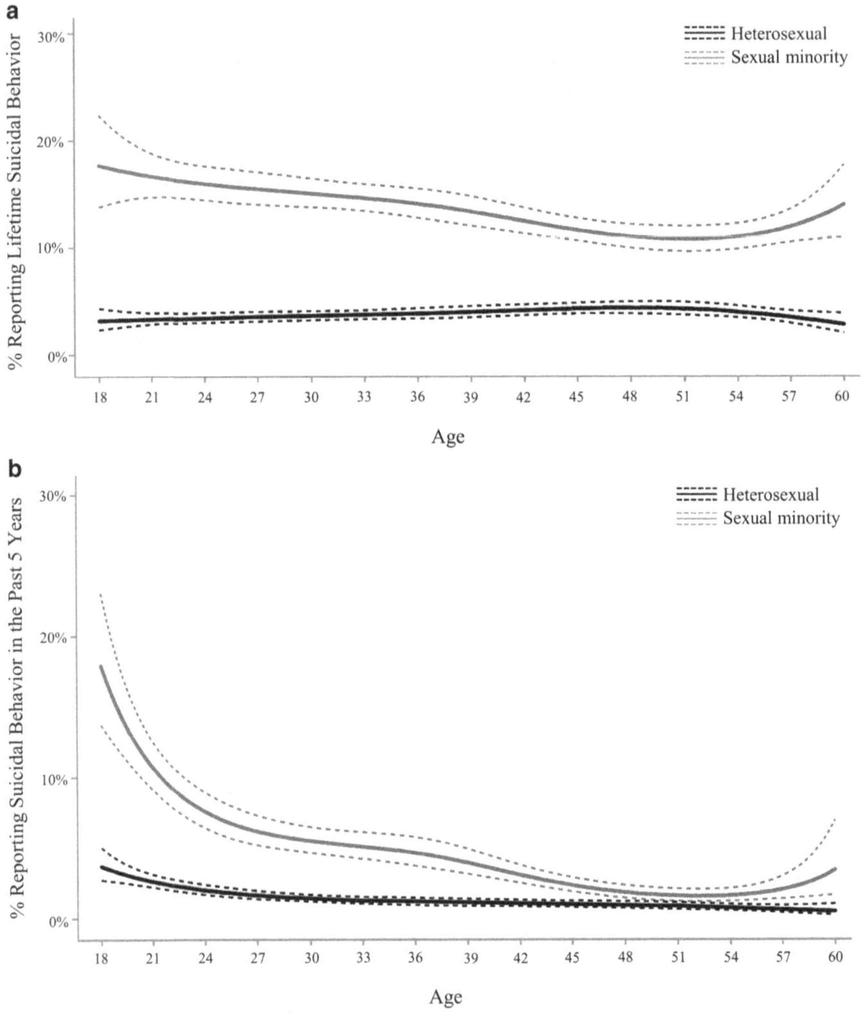

Fig. 1.1 Estimated age-varying prevalence of (**a**) lifetime and (**b**) recent suicidal behavior among heterosexual and sexual minority adults ages 18–60. Reprinted by permission from Springer Nature from Fish, J. N., Rice, C. E., Lanza, S. T., and Russell, S. T. (2019). Is young adulthood a critical period for suicidal behavior among sexual minorities? Results from a US national sample. Prevention Science, 20(3), 353–365. Copyright 2019

behavior in their life (Fig. 1.1a) and in the past 5 years (Fig. 1.1b) as a flexible function of continuous age.

Results showed that the estimated prevalence of lifetime suicidal behavior (Fig. 1.1a) among heterosexuals was around 5% across all ages, whereas the prevalence was nearly 20% among sexual minority individuals age 18 years. Among sexual minority individuals, the percent reporting suicidal behavior decreased with age, but sexual minority adults of all ages were at significantly higher odds of lifetime suicidal behavior relative to heterosexual adults. The prevalence of suicidal behavior in the past 5 years (Fig. 1.1b) was significantly higher among sexual minority adults ages 18–50 compared to heterosexual adults but was not statistically different in middle adulthood (as indicated by overlapping confidence intervals).

This study also examined discrimination as a potential mechanism for the large disparities in young adulthood by focusing on sexual minority adults only. TVEM was used to examine recent suicidal behavior, among this smaller sample of sexual minority adults, as a function of self-reported anti-LGB discrimination (coded 1 for any anti-LGB discrimination in their lifetime and 0 for none). Among sexual minority adults, the experience of anti-LGB discrimination was significantly associated with higher odds of suicidal behavior among those who are age 18–25 years, as shown by confidence intervals that do not overlap with 1.0 (Fig. 4 of the original study, reproduced here as Fig. 1.2). This association was strongest among sexual minority adults at age 18, with an odds ratio of approximately 10. In other words, among sexual minority adults age 18 years, those reporting anti-LGB discrimination had 10 times higher odds of recent suicidal behavior than those not reporting discrimination. This association weakened with age and was statistically significant through age 26. Among sexual minority adults ages 27–60, there was no significant association between anti-LGB discrimination and suicidal behavior.

The precise age ranges at which an association is significant or nonsignificant must be interpreted with caution, as age-specific confidence intervals depend on numerous factors, including the number of participants at each age and the changing base prevalence across age. Yet, taken together, this information may assist in designing interventions aimed at mitigating the risk for suicidal behavior associated with sexual minority status. In particular, the use of TVEM revealed nuanced age trends in suicidal behavior, disparities, and the link between risk factors (e.g., LGB discrimination) and suicidal behavior. Taken together, TVEM allowed these investigators to refine existing knowledge about the heightened risk for suicidal behavior among sexual minority adults by providing nuanced information across age thus informing optimal timing of suicide preventive interventions.

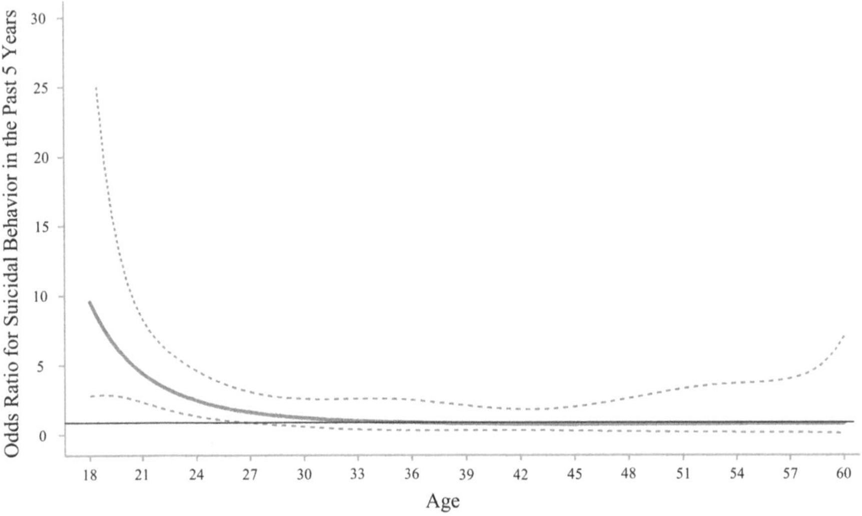

Fig. 1.2 Estimated age-varying odds ratio reflecting change in odds of recent suicidal behavior as a function of lifetime reports of anti-LGB discrimination among sexual minority adults ages 18–60 (traditional OR = 2.26, 95% CI = 1.61–3.18). Ages at which 95% confidence interval does not include the value of OR = 1.00 (shown as a horizontal line) indicate a statistically significant association. Reprinted by permission from Springer Nature from Reprinted by permission from Springer Nature from Fish, J. N., Rice, C. E., Lanza, S. T., and Russell, S. T. (2019). Is young adulthood a critical period for suicidal behavior among sexual minorities? Results from a US national sample. Prevention Science, 20(3), 359. Copyright 2019

1.4 Broader Application of TVEM in Social, Behavioral, and Health Research

Quantitative methods for analyzing data are continually advancing. We have experienced a rapid evolution of new methods for analyzing longitudinal data over the past few decades, fueled in large part by increasing capacity of personal computers to perform intensive computation needed, for example, to estimate latent variable models. Such models have become part of today's foundational methods for analyzing data, including structural equation modeling (Bollen, 1989; Little, 2013), latent growth curve modeling (Bollen & Curran, 2006; Meredith & Tisak, 1990), mediation analysis (Mackinnon, 2008), latent class and latent transition analysis (Collins & Lanza, 2010), and group-based trajectory modeling (Nagin, 2005; Nagin, Jones, Passos, & Tremblay, 2018). These models have been adopted widely because they answer important, new research questions that advance our understanding of important phenomena.

We argue that TVEM is a conceptual framework that, although arguably less complex and computationally burdensome than other approaches (e.g., latent variable modeling, Bayesian modeling), can be used to address a wide range of important research questions about how humans develop over time; the heterogeneity of people's experiences, behaviors, and outcomes as a function of historical time or age; the dynamic environment humans experience in daily life and its moment-to-moment implications; and the natural strengthening or weakening of an intervention's effect over time. As a statistical tool, when applied to existing data, TVEM can reveal valuable new information and allow researchers to address questions that previously could not be answered.

Findings based on TVEM can most certainly be useful to *researchers*. For example, epidemiologists may wish to examine nuanced age trends in the prevalence of disease or disorder, and how those trends differ across population subgroups (e.g., Vasilenko, Evans-Polce, & Lanza, 2017).

TVEM could be used to examine historical trends that would be of great interest to *policy-makers*. For example, historical trends in the perceived risk of regular use of a particular drug could be examined and used to explore the link over time between risk perceptions and behaviors (e.g., Lanza, Vasilenko, & Russell, 2016). Further investigations could examine the association between constructs such as local availability of drugs and individuals' use of drugs as a function of age and/or historical time, with the goal of identifying the potential impact of policy changes on the targeted behavior.

Practitioners may be interested in TVEM findings to understand the time-varying effect of a clinical intervention on a treatment population. Treatment effects may be examined as effecting change on an outcome over the course of treatment, ideally compared to a control group, as well as effecting change on links between core conditions such as anxiety and depressive symptoms (e.g., Wright, Hallquist, Swartz, Frank, & Cyranowski, 2014).

1.5 Structure of This Book

New empirical analyses using existing datasets were conducted to facilitate our presentation of concepts in the remaining chapters. Table 1.2 summarizes the empirical datasets and dependent variables analyzed in each chapter.

The remainder of the book is organized as follows. In Chap. 2 we present practical information on conducting TVEM in one's research. We guide the reader through the specification and interpretation in TVEM with a continuous dependent variable. Empirical results are based on analyses using data from the National Longitudinal Study of Adolescent to Adult Health (Add Health; Harris, 2013; Harris et al., 2019). The continuous variable, depressive symptoms, is modeled as a function of age, with associations allowed to vary flexibly across age throughout adolescence. We walk the reader through the features of datasets required for TVEM and discuss structuring the dataset, specifying models in SAS, centering and coding the time metric, and deciding when to estimate coefficients as time-varying or time-invariant. We also discuss the inclusion of statistical covariates and moderators of time-varying effects.

Table 1.2 Summary of new empirical analyses conducted for didactic purposes that are presented throughout this volume

Chapter	Dataset	Time variable	Data structure	Outcome type	Outcome construct
2	National Longitudinal Study of Adolescent to Adult Health (Add Health; Harris, 2013; Harris et al., 2019)	Age	Panel data	Continuous	Depressive symptoms
3	National Epidemiologic Survey on Alcohol and Related Conditions—III (NESARC-III; Grant et al., 2014)	Age	Cross-sectional	Binary	High blood pressure/ hypertension
		Age	Cross-sectional	Count	Number of drinks
4	National Epidemiologic Survey on alcohol and related conditions—III (NESARC-III)	Age	Cross-sectional	Binary	Generalized anxiety disorder
5	Monitoring the Future (MTF; Johnston et al., 2014; Miech et al., 2020)	Historical year	Repeated cross-sectional	Binary	Past 30-day smoking
6	Family Life Optimizing Well-Being (FLOW; Fosco & Lydon-Staley, 2019)	Real-time	Daily diary data	Continuous	Interparental conflict

In this chapter, we also present the technical details of model estimation in TVEM. Material covered in this chapter includes approaches to model estimation, model selection (including choosing the optimal level of complexity of coefficient functions to represent the data), adjusting standard errors when observations are not independent, and conducting weighted estimation in TVEM. This chapter also shows sample write-ups of empirical results as might be included in a manuscript.

Chapter 3 discusses extensions of TVEM for binary and count outcomes. We present logistic TVEM for binary dependent variables and Poisson TVEM for count dependent variables, focusing on the interpretation of time-varying coefficients in these frameworks. We briefly present an empirical example estimating the age-varying prevalence of high blood pressure/hypertension and examine the age-varying association between demographic characteristics (e.g., sex, racial/ethnic group, and their interaction) and high blood pressure/hypertension. To demonstrate Poisson TVEM, we present an empirical example estimating the age-varying mean number of drinks consumed during a typical drinking occasion and the age-varying association between demographic characteristics and number of drinks. This chapter also shows a sample write-up of empirical results as might be included in a manuscript.

Chapters 4, 5, and 6 present three empirical studies, each demonstrating a different metric of time. Chapter 4 examines developmental change across age, Chap. 5 models shifts to associations across historical time, and Chap. 6 examines systematic change across real-time (in this case, across days). Each chapter is designed to be similar to an empirical paper that one might write for a peer-reviewed journal, albeit with more detail on the method presented here to help readers embark on similar studies in their own research. Specifically, in each chapter we include a description of the data structure used, present the mathematical models that are estimated, and provide the SAS syntax used to estimate these models (for a more thorough explanation of data requirements, model estimation, and model selection, see Chaps. 2 and 3). An extensive list of published empirical studies that used TVEM to address questions in the social, behavioral, and health sciences can be found on the companion website for this book (https://prevention.psu.edu/books/tvem/), including a manuscript that demonstrates the application of TVEM to examine marijuana use behavior using three conceptualizations of time: age, historical time, and time relative to an event (Lanza et al., 2016).

Chapter 4 introduces readers to the use of TVEM to estimate associations that vary as a function of age. Tests of age-varying associations can include (a) tests of how associations change with development, as people age in longitudinal studies or (b) tests of how associations differ between people of different ages in a cross-sectional study. We present an empirical example of the latter, estimating an age-varying association using data from NESARC-III, a large, nationally representative, cross-sectional sample of adults. Numerous published manuscripts have used TVEM to examine age-varying associations (e.g., Kuhfeld, Gershoff, & Paschall, 2018; Lanza, Russell, & Braymiller, 2017; Linden-Carmichael, Vasilenko, Lanza, & Maggs, 2017; Vasilenko, 2017).

Chapter 5 discusses the use of TVEM to investigate historical change in prevalence of health-related behavior and time-varying associations of factors that may be driving such change. This empirical example demonstrates historical shifts in the prevalence of cigarette smoking from 1990 to 2017 and the time-varying associations of individual characteristics with this behavior using repeated cross-sectional data from the MTF data. We also discuss how other data sources (e.g., data on federal policy changes, public health awareness campaigns) could be integrated to examine their time-varying associations with health outcomes. Several previous studies have used TVEM to examine change across historical time (e.g., Lanza, Vasilenko, Dziak, & Butera, 2015; Terry-McElrath, O'Malley, Patrick, & Miech, 2017).

Chapter 6 discusses the use of TVEM for examining time-varying associations in ILD, such as ILD generated from studies using wearable devices, mobile phone surveys (as in ecological momentary assessment), social media (Facebook, Twitter), and global positioning systems (GPS). Here, we present an empirical example using data from an electronic daily diary study of two-parent families with an adolescent between 13 and 16 years of age. Both parents and the adolescent participated in a 21-day study of emotion and family functioning. We present an application of TVEM where time is centered at the occurrence of a family event, specifically the first parent-reported conflict event during the study. Interparental conflict is modeled as a nonparametric function of time relative to the conflict event in order to examine anticipatory anger and recovery from the event. A number of prior studies have applied TVEM to examine questions about dynamic constructs in real-time using ILD (e.g., Maher & Dunton, 2020; Mason et al., 2015; Shiyko, Burkhalter, Li, & Park, 2014; Vasilenko et al., 2014).

Finally, in Chap. 7, we focus on the enormous potential TVEM holds for application in the behavioral, social, and health sciences. This includes a discussion of the many ways to conceive of "time" in TVEM, each enabling researchers to empirically address new research questions and inform the way we think about theory. We then compare TVEM to other analytic approaches, with a focus on similarities and differences between TVEM and multilevel modeling (and the special case of growth curve modeling) for longitudinal data. We also comment briefly on missing data, statistical power analysis, and sample size requirements. We conclude with a brief summary of the active methodological work on TVEM and future methodological research that would further expand the use of TVEM in social, behavioral, and health sciences.

References

Bollen, K. A. (1989). *Structural equation modeling with latent constructs*. Wiley-Interscience.

Bollen, K. A., & Curran, P. J. (2006). *Latent curve models: A structural equation perspective* (Vol. 467). Hoboken, NJ: John Wiley & Sons.

Collins, L. M., & Lanza, S. T. (2010). *Latent class and latent transition analysis: With applications in the social, behavioral, and health sciences*. John Wiley & Sons.

Fish, J. N., Rice, C. E., Lanza, S. T., & Russell, S. T. (2019). Is young adulthood a critical period for suicidal behavior among sexual minorities? Results from a US national sample. *Prevention Science, 20*(3), 353–365.

Fosco, G. M., & Lydon-Staley, D. M. (2019). A within-family examination of interparental conflict, cognitive appraisals, and adolescent mood and well-being. *Child Development, 90*(4), e421–e436.

Grant, B. F., Chu, A., Sigman, R., Amsbary, M., Kali, J., Sugawara, Y., Jiao, R., Ren, W., & Goldstein, R. (2014). *Source and accuracy statement: National Epidemiologic Survey on Alcohol and Related Conditions-III (NESARC-III)* (pp. 1–125). National Institute on Alcohol Abuse and Alcoholism.

Harris, K. M. (2013). *The Add Health study: Design and accomplishments*. Carolina Population Center, University of North Carolina at Chapel Hill.

Harris, K. M., Halpern, C. T., Whitsel, E. A., Hussey, J. M., Killeya-Jones, L. A., Tabor, J., & Dean, S. C. (2019). Cohort profile: The national longitudinal study of adolescent to adult health (Add Health). *International Journal of Epidemiology, 48*(5), 1415–1415.

Johnston, L. D., O'Malley, P. M., Bachman, J. G., Schulenberg, J. E., & Miech, R. A. (2014). *Monitoring the Future: National survey results on drug use, 1975–2013: Volume I, secondary school students*. Institute for Social Research, University of Michigan.

Kuhfeld, M., Gershoff, E., & Paschall, K. (2018). The development of racial/ethnic and socioeconomic achievement gaps during the school years. *Journal of Applied Developmental Psychology, 57*, 62–73.

Lanza, S. T., Russell, M. A., & Braymiller, J. L. (2017). Emergence of electronic cigarette use in US adolescents and the link to traditional cigarette use. *Addictive Behaviors, 67*, 38–43.

Lanza, S. T., Vasilenko, S. A., Dziak, J. J., & Butera, N. M. (2015). Trends among US high school seniors in recent marijuana use and associations with other substances: 1976–2013. *Journal of Adolescent Health, 57*(2), 198–204.

Lanza, S. T., Vasilenko, S. A., & Russell, M. A. (2016). Time-varying effect modeling to address new questions in behavioral research: Examples in marijuana use. *Psychology of Addictive Behaviors, 30*(8), 939–954.

Linden-Carmichael, A. N., Vasilenko, S. A., Lanza, S. T., & Maggs, J. L. (2017). High-intensity drinking versus heavy episodic drinking: Prevalence rates and relative odds of alcohol use disorder across adulthood. *Alcoholism: Clinical and Experimental Research, 41*(10), 1754–1759.

Little, T. D. (2013). *Longitudinal structural equation modeling*. Guilford Press.

MacKinnon, D. (2008). *Intoduction to statistical mediation analysis*. Taylor &Francis Group.

Maher, J. P., & Dunton, G. F. (2020). Within-day time-varying associations between motivation and movement-related behaviors in older adults. *Psychology of Sport and Exercise, 47*, 101522.

Mason, M., Mennis, J., Way, T., Lanza, S., Russell, M., & Zaharakis, N. (2015). Time-varying effects of a text-based smoking cessation intervention for urban adolescents. *Drug and Alcohol Dependence, 157*, 99–105.

Meredith, W., & Tisak, J. (1990). Latent curve analysis. *Psychometrika, 55*(1), 107–122.

Miech, R., Johnston, L., O'Malley, P., Bachman, J., Schulenberg, J., & Patrick, M. (2020). *Monitoring the future national survey results on drug use, 1975–2019: Volume I, Secondary school students*. Institute for Social Research, The University of Michigan.

Nagin, D. S. (2005). *Group-based modeling of development*. Harvard University Press.

Nagin, D. S., Jones, B. L., Passos, V. L., & Tremblay, R. E. (2018). Group-based multi-trajectory modeling. *Statistical Methods in Medical Research, 27*(7), 2015–2023.

Shiyko, M. P., Burkhalter, J., Li, R., & Park, B. J. (2014). Modeling nonlinear time-dependent treatment effects: An application of the generalized time-varying effect model (TVEM). *Journal of Consulting and Clinical Psychology, 82*(5), 760–772.

Terry-McElrath, Y. M., O'Malley, P. M., Patrick, M. E., & Miech, R. A. (2017). Risk is still relevant: Time-varying associations between perceived risk and marijuana use among US 12th grade students from 1991 to 2016. *Addictive Behaviors, 74*, 13–19.

Vasilenko, S. A. (2017). Age-varying associations between nonmarital sexual behavior and depressive symptoms across adolescence and young adulthood. *Developmental Psychology, 53*(2), 366–378.

Vasilenko, S. A., Evans-Polce, R. J., & Lanza, S. T. (2017). Age trends in rates of substance use disorders across ages 18–90: Differences by gender and race/ethnicity. *Drug and Alcohol Dependence, 180*, 260–264.

Vasilenko, S. A., Piper, M. E., Lanza, S. T., Liu, X., Yang, J., & Li, R. (2014). Time-varying processes involved in smoking lapse in a randomized trial of smoking cessation therapies. *Nicotine & Tobacco Research, 16*(Suppl_2), S135–S143.

Wright, A. G., Hallquist, M. N., Swartz, H. A., Frank, E., & Cyranowski, J. M. (2014). Treating co-occurring depression and anxiety: Modeling the dynamics of psychopathology and psychotherapy using the time-varying effect model. *Journal of Consulting and Clinical Psychology, 82*(5), 839–853.

Chapter 2
Specifying, Estimating, and Interpreting Time-Varying Effect Models

In any statistical analysis, a researcher must align three crucial elements: (1) a *research question*, (2) *data* that will allow one to address the question, and (3) a *statistical model* that, when applied to the data at hand, will allow a test of the research question. Chapter 1 oriented the reader to the types of research questions that can be addressed with time-varying effect modeling (TVEM). Chapter 2 will walk through the data considerations for TVEM and a step-by-step guide for how to conduct TVEM. This chapter is divided into four sections. First, we discuss data requirements for TVEM. Second, we present technical details on model estimation and model selection. Third, we walk through the specification of four statistical models, building on the hypothetical example raised in Chap. 1 (in the section titled "TVEM as a Simple Extension of Linear Regression"), supposing one is interested in age-varying sex differences in career satisfaction. Continuing with our hypothetical example, these models include the following:

- **Model 1:** An intercept-only TVEM (e.g., overall mean career satisfaction across age);
- **Model 2:** Estimating the mean of an outcome as a function of a single covariate of interest (e.g., age-varying association between sex and career satisfaction);
- **Model 3:** An extension of Model 2 that incorporates an additional covariate (e.g., age-varying association between sex and career satisfaction holding constant, or controlling for, college degree attainment); and
- **Model 4:** A statistical moderation analysis that includes an interaction term (e.g., to assess how an age-varying sex difference in career satisfaction differs, across age, as a function of college degree attainment).

For each model, we describe the mathematical model, the variables included in the analysis, how to specify the model in SAS, and how to interpret the parameter estimates (i.e., coefficient functions). Fourth, we turn to an empirical example on depressive symptoms across age, walking the reader through data preparation, model specification, model selection, and interpretation of the results. We conclude

S. T. Lanza, A. N. Linden-Carmichael, *Time-Varying Effect Modeling for the Behavioral, Social, and Health Sciences*,
https://doi.org/10.1007/978-3-030-70944-0_2

the chapter with a brief sample results section for a manuscript based on the depressive symptoms example. We note that this entire chapter focuses on modeling an outcome with a continuous distribution. Generalized TVEM, specifically for a binary or count outcome, is presented in Chap. 3.

2.1 Data Considerations

2.1.1 Data Coverage Across Time

Because TVEM estimates associations between variables across continuous time, researchers need to have data with adequate *coverage across the span of time being studied*. For example, suppose one is interested in studying sexual behavior across ages 14–32 using longitudinal panel data. If the study design sampled every participant at only ages 14, 22, and 32, then there would be significant gaps in the coverage of age, and TVEM might not be an appropriate method. A better design to study this age range using longitudinal panel data would be a cohort-sequential design, where, for example, participants at Wave 1 were of varying ages across adolescence, providing a similar number of observations at, say, ages 15 and 30 years. This has implications for statistical power potentially varying across time, as discussed in Chap. 7. However, the width of confidence intervals in TVEM varies with time, and thus, all else being equal, confidence intervals for the coefficients will be wider at times when data are sparser. Thus, the researcher can rest assured that any interpolation of coefficients at times with little data will correspond to greater uncertainty, as reflected in wider confidence intervals.

2.1.2 Types of Data That Can be Analyzed in TVEM

Coverage of the time axis can be achieved with several types of data. When *intensive longitudinal data* (ILD), such as ecological momentary assessments (EMA), are used, each person may have many measurement occasions across the time axis. Chapter 6 presents an analysis of daily diary data where individuals have somewhat intensive assessments, and time is centered at a self-reported conflict event between a couple. In this example, all participants provided data on multiple days prior to and following the event, providing adequate coverage. On the other extreme, *cross-sectional data* can be used to examine age-varying effects with TVEM if there are enough people in the study assessed at different ages. Chapter 4 presents an analysis of cross-sectional data where individuals ranged in age from 18–65. There were many individuals in the large dataset at various ages, providing excellent coverage across the entire age range. As in any study of development, researchers need to think carefully about whether differences observed are due to age or whether they could be caused by cohort effects. This is particularly problematic when using cross-sectional data or panel data with a wide age range and few measurement occasions.

Longitudinal panel data may be appropriate for TVEM if there are many assessments per person (e.g., everyone in the study was assessed every fall and spring throughout middle and high school) or if a cohort-sequential design, also referred to as an accelerated longitudinal design, were employed. The empirical example presented later in this chapter relies on data from a national study that used a cohort-sequential design in which participants were in grades 7–12 at Wave 1 and followed up at several additional time points. Another type of data that can provide good coverage over time is *repeated cross-sectional survey data*, where the same survey is administered each year to a new cohort for many years. Chapter 5 presents an analysis of this type of data, with cohorts of high school seniors reporting on the same measures across historical time from 1990–2017.

As with classic regression analysis, in TVEM the *distribution of the outcome variable* has implications for the model being specified. The standard TVEM, the focus of the current chapter, assumes that the outcome follows a Gaussian distribution (i.e., that the outcome is normally distributed). The empirical demonstration woven throughout this chapter relies on an outcome, depressive symptom score, that is assumed to follow a Gaussian distribution. TVEM has been generalized to handle both binary and count outcomes by assuming that the outcome follows a binomial or Poisson distribution, respectively (see Chap. 3 for a description of generalized TVEM). For the time being, it is sufficient to understand that the distributional assumptions made within a particular moment of time in TVEM correspond to those we must make in traditional regression analysis. If one were to use logistic regression or Poisson regression to model the association among variables at a particular time, then logistic TVEM or Poisson TVEM, respectively, would most likely be needed to estimate time-varying associations when modeling that outcome variable.

Time-varying effect models can be estimated with all of these different types of data. As with any longitudinal analysis, the measurement of any constructs assessed over time is assumed to be the same. Additionally, researchers need to be careful with the interpretations of their results when using cross-sectional or accelerated longitudinal designs. If a cross-sectional study includes individuals from a wide range of ages, it can be difficult to disentangle age effects (developmental differences) from cohort effects (differences for individuals born in different time periods). When describing these types of analyses, researchers should be careful in their interpretations and discuss the limitations inherent in these data. Despite this limitation, these types of data can give us important information when an intensive longitudinal study is not possible.

2.1.3 Preparing Data for TVEM

Four steps are needed to prepare data for conducting TVEM. First, much like data for many other longitudinal models (mixed models, generalized estimating equations), data for TVEM need to be arranged in "long" (i.e., "stacked") form, with each row of data containing information for a single person at a single time point, and a person-ID variable indicating the individual who provided data at that time point (repeated for each row of data for that person). Second, an intercept needs to be manually created in the dataset. This can be done by creating a new variable, which we often give the arbitrary label *INT*, that is equal to 1 for all records in the dataset. Third, a variable containing the value of time for each record must be included and recentered if necessary for time = 0 to have a meaning that facilitates interpretation. Throughout this book, our empirical examples center time in different ways, including birth (when examining coefficients across age; see Chap. 4), a particular year in history (when examining coefficients across historical time; see Chap. 5), and the day of first observed marital conflict event (see Chap. 6). Fourth, the coverage of observations along the time axis needs to be examined. Ideally, as mentioned above, there will be a representation of data points for the outcome (i.e., dependent variable) across the entire time axis. We note that all covariates must be coded by the analyst so that they can be treated as numeric in the analysis. For example, a binary covariate should be coded 0 or 1 for each observation, and a multinomial covariate with *m* response options should be recoded into a set of *m*-1 dummy variables, as this macro will not recode categorical variables automatically as in other SAS procedures. When interaction terms are of interest in TVEM, variables must be coded manually by taking the product of the two variables. Centering and/or standardization of continuous covariates also should be considered prior to estimating a time-varying effect model in a way similar to considering centering/standardization of covariates in traditional regression. For example, if a scale of 0–100 is used to indicate the level of stress, the expected effect of a one-unit change on an outcome may look quite trivial even if statistically significant. In cases where a covariate is on a scale with arbitrary meaning, it can be useful to standardize the covariate before estimating a model, as TVEM does not produce standardized regression coefficients.

2.2 Estimating Coefficient Functions

2.2.1 Two Approaches to Spline Estimation

A *spline* is a curve composed of connected line segments (line segments may be linear or some other parametric form such as quadratic or cubic). The points at which these lines connect (sometimes called inflection points) are called *knots*. Splines are useful because they allow a high degree of flexibility when estimating the shape of a nonlinear function. In TVEM, splines are used to represent intercepts and slopes (i.e., regression coefficients) estimated such that the nature of change across continuous time can be complex and nonlinear, and need not be specified a priori. This can add specificity to the underlying nature of change over time in outcomes and in associations, rather than only revealing a highly constrained nature of change, such as linear across time. There are various mathematical ways to estimate a spline; the two methods available in TVEM are P-spline and B-spline. Each has advantages, depending on the specific model one is estimating and with what purpose.

P-spline is short for a truncated power spline basis. This estimation technique tends to lead to smoother curves for coefficient functions than B-spline.[1] When using P-spline, the degree of complexity of each coefficient function is automatically selected by the macro. We recommend specifying around 10 knots in the macro to ensure that sufficient complexity in the curve shape can be considered (although in practice 5 knots is more than sufficient for most models). In addition to automatically selecting the optimal complexity of the curves, P-spline automatically applies robust standard errors to handle the nonindependence of repeated assessments that characterizes all longitudinal data.

When specifying a *B-spline* basis for the estimation method, model selection must be done manually. Here, model selection does not refer to deciding whether to include certain covariates; in TVEM, model selection refers to selecting the optimal number of knots in each coefficient function being estimated in a given model. In other words, if a time-varying effect model predicting an outcome from a particular set of covariates is desired, the number of knots for the intercept function and any slope functions are chosen by comparing models in terms of the *Akaike information criterion (AIC)* and *Bayesian information criterion (BIC)*. These information criteria are used for model selection in a wide variety of statistical models and work well with TVEM. They are designed to optimally balance model fit with model parsimony by penalizing the log-likelihood value, with a larger penalty corresponding to more complex curves. Models with lower AIC and/or BIC are considered to have the desired number of knots in TVEM.

[1] The reader may wonder why we explain the reason for the name "P-spline" but not the reason for the name "B-spline." When they were proposed in the 1940s, B-splines meant "basic splines," but this did NOT mean that they were simpler or easier than other kinds of splines—basic referred to the fact that they used different functions of time, which formed a geometric basis for constructing the spline. (*Basis* here means a set of functions or dimensions that you take a linear combination of, in order to make objects in a space of possible objects.) This does not provide any intuition however because any kind of spline has some kind of basis functions. Thus, it is a historical artifact. When we use the word P-splines in the TVEM macro, we use it in a slightly nonstandard way to mean penalized truncated powers of time. Others (e.g., Eilers and Marx (1996)) have used it to refer to penalized B-spline bases.

2.2.1.1 Model Selection in B-Spline Estimation

One approach to model selection is to compare the relative fit of models with all possible combinations of numbers of knots. In the simplest example, an intercept-only time-varying effect model, one could compare the relative fit of models with 1 through 5 knots and select the one with the lowest AIC and/or BIC. As another example, in a model with a time-varying intercept and time-varying coefficients for two covariates, the number of knots must be selected for each of the three coefficient functions. One could estimate and compare fit of all possible permutations; if one considers from 1 to 5 knots per function, a total of $5^3 = 125$ models would be compared, corresponding to models with knots of 1, 1, 1, knots of 1, 1, 2, and so on, all the way to a model with knots of 5, 5, 5. From these 125 models, the one with the lowest AIC and/or BIC may be selected. Clearly however as the complexity of the model specified increases, this exhaustive approach to model selection can be extremely time-intensive and tedious. In practice, this approach works well when estimating only 1 or 2 coefficient functions.

We have found the following streamlined model selection procedure to be sufficient for models involving the estimation of 3 or more coefficient functions. We recommend beginning by estimating the model corresponding to the most complex functions (i.e., the maximum number of knots) being considered. In the example involving an intercept function and two coefficient functions, this might be the model with knots of 5, 5, 5. Next, we vary the number of knots for one of the higher order functions (e.g., one of the functions corresponding to a covariate, rather than the intercept function; in models with an interaction term this would be the highest order function) and select from among that subset of models (in this case, 5 models) to determine the optimal number of knots corresponding to that function, and fix that value. Then, we vary the number of knots for the next highest order function and select from among that subset of models (in this case, another set of 5 models where the number of knots for the highest order function has been selected and set to that value). This procedure continues until we consider the number of knots for the intercept function. For this example, in contrast to comparing models with all 125 possible permutations of the number of knots, we compare, at most, $5 * 3 = 15$ models. This model-selection approach with B-spline, which is demonstrated in the fourth section of this chapter, tends to result in more fine-tuned functions (i.e., more complex functions that show more nuance/change over time) than the automatic model-selection approach implemented in P-spline.

As a general practice, one may wish to first use P-spline (with a large number of knots, e.g., 10) to gain a quick understanding of the data. A large number of knots ensures that the algorithm automatically selects a good amount of smoothness. This conveys the general features of coefficient functions being estimated. Then, one can switch to B-spline to fine-tune the analysis; in other words, this allows manual selection of the optimal number of knots, allowing one to see the proper level of detail in the time-varying coefficients being modeled. Importantly, there is no information contained in the output from P-spline that guides the number of knots to specify when switching to B-spline; rather, the model selection procedure in

B-spline should proceed independently. The goal of an initial P-spline estimation is simply to gain insight into the data; in many cases, P-spline estimation is sufficient for publishing results. Reasons one may wish to proceed to B-spline estimation despite the added requirement of conducting model selection manually include the following:

1. Typically, the model selection procedure with B-spline results in curves that are more complex and nuanced than the curves produced using P-spline estimation, as B-spline is more sensitive to curve fluctuations.
2. B-spline can be used for weighted analyses. In this case, one may wish to skip the preliminary step of using P-spline and conduct all analyses using B-spline with weights.
3. B-spline can accommodate random effects to handle nonindependence of repeated assessments, which may be preferred to the robust standard errors produced in P-spline estimation to address this nonindependence.

2.2.2 Addressing Nonindependence of Repeated Assessments

As in any longitudinal data analysis, it is important to consider how to handle nonindependence of repeated assessments. The %TVEM macro can model within-subject correlation, which is necessary to address when analyzing repeated-measures data, using two different approaches that are commonly used in other models: robust standard errors (i.e., "sandwich" standard errors) and random effects. The *robust standard errors* approach calculates the estimates as though the observations were independent and then adjusts the standard errors to account for the fact that they are not. This method is automatically used with P-spline estimation, and thus the user need not specify anything other than ensuring that the "ID" variable is the one indicating the level of clustering for which to adjust. The *random effects* approach is available with B-spline estimation in the %TVEM macro and requires that the user specify whether to estimate no random effects, a random intercept, or a random intercept and a random slope. Each random effect specified in the model adds a term to the model to account for the different characteristics of each individual. Specifying no random effects treats all observations as independent. Specifying a random intercept-only treats all observations within the same person as equally correlated. Specifying a random intercept and a random slope automatically allows an individual's observations that are closer in time to be more highly correlated than those spaced further apart in time. This last specification is typically the most plausible, but the model may fail to converge due to its complexity. If convergence of a random intercept and a random slope is not possible, we recommend specifying a random intercept-only if one is analyzing repeated-measures data. We refer readers to Section 7 of the TVEM users' guide (Li et al., 2017) for technical detail on P-spline estimation, B-spline estimation, and random effects in TVEM.

Just as the coefficients are estimated as a function of time, so are the corresponding standard errors. Rather than calculating and interpreting a p-value at a particular moment in time, TVEM results are plotted in figures with the point estimate of the coefficient and corresponding 95% confidence interval across the range of time. In TVEM, all confidence bands for coefficient functions are *pointwise confidence bands*, meaning that, at any specific value of t, the confidence interval covers the corresponding true value of the regression coefficient with confidence 0.95. Pointwise confidence bands do not correct for multiple comparisons and thus do not imply joint confidence over all time points together, but rather enable researchers to interpret confidence intervals at particular values of t.[2]

This information presents interesting opportunities for researchers to draw inferences from their findings. For example, an association may be statistically significant (as indicated by confidence intervals that do not include the value of 0) at one specific time point but may be nonsignificant at other times. Thus, one of the first ways to interpret a coefficient function is to describe the times at which the coefficient is statistically significantly different from 0 and the times at which it is not significant. In other words, rather than evaluating whether a covariate is significantly associated with an outcome (overall, as in classic regression analysis), we can evaluate *times at which* a covariate is significantly associated with the outcome.

2.2.3 TVEM Specification in SAS

A user-friendly SAS macro has been created to easily *specify a time-varying effect model in SAS*. The %TVEM macro is designed to run on SAS version 9.2 or higher and requires that one's SAS install includes SAS/IML and SAS/STAT (which is typically included in SAS licenses). The users' guide (Li et al., 2017) provides details on how to install and run the macro. Table 2.1 lists all arguments, both required and optional, defined in the macro, along with a brief description of their functionality. We present this table to give the reader a sense of the capabilities of current software for conducting TVEM. Throughout the remainder of this book, the specific SAS syntax used to conduct each empirical analysis will be presented. Table 2.1 serves as a reference to that syntax. Note that SAS is not case sensitive in its variable names or arguments.

The handling of *missing data in TVEM* is an important area of future research, and the issue is somewhat complex. The %TVEM macro uses all available data from each individual at each time point. For specific observations (i.e., rows of data in the "long" format) at which either the outcome or any covariates in a model are missing, that observation is automatically excluded from the analysis. However,

[2] This is in contrast to simultaneous confidence bands, which are constructed such that the probability that the confidence intervals at every point across t contain their true values simultaneously is 0.95. In practice, simultaneous bands with the same coverage probability as pointwise confidence bands would be much wider.

Table 2.1 Brief summary of %TVEM SAS macro arguments

Argument	Functionality
Required	
data	Name of analysis dataset (long format; one record per assessment)
dist	Distribution of outcome variable (options: normal, logistic, or Poisson)
id	Unique numeric ID for each unit of analysis, typically an individual
time	Name of variable containing indicator of time of each assessment
dv	Dependent variable (i.e., outcome)
tvary_effect	Covariates specified to have time-varying coefficient, treated as numeric
method	Estimation method (options: P-spline or B-spline)
knots	Number of knots corresponding to each time-varying coefficient
Optional	
degree	Degree of polynomial used between curve knots (options: 1, 2, or 3 (default))
evenly	Distributes knots evenly across quintiles of observations or across time range
invar_effect	Covariates specified to have time-invariant coefficient
output_ prefix	Specifies where output datasets are saved
outfilename	Generates a .Csv file containing data for plotting in other software programs
plot	Type of plots to be generated (options: full, simple, or none)
plot_scale	Number of points to be plotted in coefficient functions
random	Method for estimating within-subject correlation (options: none, intercept, or slope)
stderr	Method used to calculate standard errors (options: robust or standard)

TVEM does not remove those individuals from the dataset entirely but retains any specific observations with no missing data (i.e., TVEM does not use casewise deletion). The topic of missing data is revisited in Chap. 7.

An important feature of TVEM is that it does not make strong *model assumptions*, specifically about the form of change in coefficients across time. TVEM can be considered nonparametric modeling, requiring no constraints on shapes of coefficient functions. Instead, shapes are estimated from the available data; the only assumption is that changes with time happen gradually and in a smooth way. More specifically, TVEM makes the following assumptions: (1) for a given time, or point on the coefficient function, associations among variables are assumed to be linear—the linearity assumption in multiple regression analysis holds in TVEM *within a particular time*; (2) all coefficient functions are smooth functions across time, but discontinuities can be estimated if one prespecifies them to occur at a particular common time (e.g., at age 21, when alcohol use becomes legal in the United States) or when a particular event occurs (e.g., upon the transition from middle school to high school; upon quitting smoking; at a historical year when the legalization of a substance changed); and (3) any specified random effects are normally distributed and independent.

This flexibility lends itself well to many analyses of ILD where the outcome and associations of covariates may vary systematically with time, for example in an EMA study of adults who quit smoking and are assessed multiple times per day for several weeks. With TVEM, there is no need to assume that growth occurs as a parametric function of time (i.e., linear, quadratic) or that the effects of covariates are constant over time. Instead, direction and strength of association are estimated over time using EMA data from multiple individuals (i.e., regression coefficients can change with time). This approach accommodates variability across individuals in timing and spacing of observations, which is inherent in EMA studies that randomly prompt participants.

2.2.4 *Weighted Analysis in TVEM*

A separate SAS macro, %WeightedTVEM, has been developed to estimate time-varying effect models that accommodate *sample weights and clustering*. Many complex datasets exist that involve clustering (e.g., students nested within schools) and/or sample weights (e.g., participants represent different numbers of population members due to a design involving systematically unequally probabilities of selection, such as oversampling of a particular racial/ethnic group). By incorporating sample weights in an analysis, findings better represent the population about which inferences are drawn. The %TVEM macro described above does not accommodate sample weights or clustering, other than the clustering of repeated observations within individuals. The weighted macro can accommodate continuous and binary outcomes, but at this writing the macro does not support count outcomes. B-spline estimation is used, and robust standard errors are provided (as opposed to random effects). These standard errors are constructed using Taylor linearization, as in generalized estimating equations (GEEs; Liang & Zeger, 1986). Technical details about estimation in %WeightedTVEM can be found in the corresponding users' guide (Dziak, Li, & Wagner, 2017).

As with most GEE procedures, the weighted TVEM macro allows only a single level of nesting to be explicitly specified. In cases where there are multiple levels of clustering, for example, repeated measures of individuals who are nested within schools, it is recommended that users specify the highest level of clustering (school) as GEE does not require a correct specification of within-cluster correlation in order to obtain unbiased estimates. Further, the AIC and BIC in a weighted analysis are based on the pseudolikelihood function rather than the log-likelihood function, but still can be used to guide model selection. Section 3 of the users' guide (Dziak et al., 2017) includes a detailed discussion of these issues.

2.3 Model Specification: A Progression Through Four Models

In this section, we walk readers through a progression of models with increasing complexity. In this hypothetical example, we examine career satisfaction, a continuous scale score with good psychometric properties, as our outcome variable. The data are from a cross-sectional study of 5000 adult full-time employees across ages 25–65, and there is good coverage of data across the age range (e.g., the distribution of age in the sample is relatively uniform). We are interested in specifying models that (Model 1) reveal the estimated age trend in career satisfaction; (Model 2) examine the direction and size of sex differences in career satisfaction as a function of age by including sex as a covariate; (Model 3) estimate the direction and size of sex differences in career satisfaction as a function of age, controlling for whether the individuals attained a college degree; and (Model 4) examine age-varying moderation of the association between sex and career satisfaction by college degree attainment. For each model, we walk the reader through the mathematical model that is specified to address the question, describe the interpretation of the model parameters, summarize variables required in the analysis, and present SAS syntax to estimate the model. The dataset contains the following seven variables for each individual *i*:

- Unique participant id (*CASEID*),
- Participant's age, which represents "time" in these models (*AGE*),
- Career satisfaction (*SAT*),
- Vector of 1's to specify the intercept (*INT*),
- Indicator of participant's sex, coded female = 0 and male = 1 (*SEX*),
- Indicator of whether participant completed a 4-year college degree, coded no = 0 and yes = 1 (*COLLEGE*), and
- Indicator derived by taking the product of SEX by COLLEGE (*SEX_COLLEGE*).

2.3.1 Model 1: Intercept-Only TVEM

In this model, we specify an intercept-Only TVEM to estimate the mean career satisfaction across continuous age, as follows:

$$SAT_i = \beta_0\left(t\right) + \epsilon_i,$$

where SAT_i represents the career satisfaction score for individual *i*, $\beta_0(t)$ is the intercept function, which represents the estimated mean career satisfaction score as a continuous function across ages 25–65, and the error term, ϵ_i, reflects individual *i*'s deviation from that curve (i.e., the difference between their observed and expected career satisfaction for an adult of their specific age). The variables needed to estimate this model include *CASEID*, *AGE*, *SAT*, and *INT*.

To estimate this model, we specified a %TVEM macro statement in SAS:

```
%TVEM(
data = career_chapter2a,
dist = normal,
id = caseid,
time = age,
dv = sat,
tvary_effect = int,
method = P-spline,
knots = 10);
```

The **data** statement is the name of our analysis dataset, which in the case of cross-sectional data has one record per person (i.e., a standard rectangular dataset). Because the outcome is continuous, we specify the distribution to be "normal" for our **dist** statement. The **id** statement refers to the unique participant ID variable. **Time** refers to how we specify time on the *x*-axis; in this case, time is considered participants' age, which is stored in the variable *AGE*. We note that this variable can be a real number, for example, the age variable could be integers from 18 to 65 or values could have greater precision, such as age = 45.62. Readers are encouraged to retain higher levels of precision when available, but coarser measurement can be used when necessary. We note that the minimum and maximum values of age are not specified, rather the program detects the age range and automatically presents coefficient functions across those values. **DV** is the outcome of interest; here, our outcome is a scale score for career satisfaction, labeled as *SAT*. Because this simple model evaluates only the estimated prevalence of the dependent variable (*SAT*) across age, our **tvary_effect** will include only the intercept. We have already created a variable in our dataset (called *INT*) which is equal to 1 for all rows of data. Because only one variable is specified in the **tvary_effect** statement, only one coefficient function will be estimated—in this case, an intercept function.

The **method** argument is where users specify whether the model should be fit using B-spline or P-spline estimation. In this hypothetical example, the data are not weighted and we are interested in running our first model to these data thus we specify P-spline. It is possible to subsequently re-specify the model using B-spline in order to fine-tune the curve, possibly revealing more nuance in its shape. Because we have specified P-spline, our **knots** statement refers to the number of knots to be included (which is specified here as 10). The P-spline algorithm automatically selects the appropriate amount of smoothing, so the user need not perform model selection.

2.3.2 *Model 2: TVEM With a Main Effect*

In this model, we specify a main-effects TVEM to estimate the sex difference in career satisfaction across continuous age (i.e., an age-varying sex difference in career satisfaction), as follows:

$$SAT_i = \beta_0(t) + \beta_1(t)SEX_i + \epsilon_i,$$

where SAT_i represents the career satisfaction score for individual i, SEX_i indicates individual i's sex, $\beta_0(t)$ is the intercept function, which now represents the estimated mean career satisfaction score as a continuous function across ages 25–65 *for female adults* (i.e., where $SEX = 0$), $\beta_1(t)$ is the coefficient function for *SEX*, representing the estimated increase (or decrease) in career satisfaction for male compared to female adults across ages 25–65, and the error term, ϵ_i, reflects individual i's deviation from their expected career satisfaction (i.e., the difference between their observed and expected career satisfaction for an adult of their specific age and sex. The variables needed to estimate this model include *CASEID*, *AGE*, *SAT*, *INT*, and *SEX*.

To estimate this model, we specified a %TVEM macro statement in SAS.

```
%TVEM(
data = career_chapter2a,
dist = normal,
id = caseid,
time = age,
dv = sat,
tvary_effect = int sex,
method = P-spline,
knots = 10 10);
```

The arguments are nearly identical to those in Model 1, with the following exceptions. Because this model is to estimate the main effect of sex, our **tvary_effect** now includes two variables: *int* and *sex*. Two coefficient functions will be estimated—in this case, an intercept function and a slope function, also referred to as a coefficient function for *sex*. Because we are now estimating two coefficient functions, which may have different amounts of complexity in the function across age, our **knots** statement refers to the maximum number of knots (specifically, interior knots) to be considered for each. We list 10 knots for each; the order of the values listed in the **knots** statement corresponds to the order of the variables listed in the **tvary_effect** argument. The P-spline algorithm automatically selects the optimal complexity for both coefficient functions.

2.3.3 Model 3: TVEM With a Statistical Control Variable

Building on Model 2, we now add college degree attainment as a statistical control variable. This allows us to interpret the association between sex and career satisfaction, controlling for college degree attainment. Note that more than one control variable may be included in a model simultaneously, and they can comprise any combination of binary and continuous variables. Centering of control variables is important to consider, as it will determine the appropriate interpretation of the intercept function. This issue is identical to how one interprets an intercept in standard linear regression when control variables are included.

To control for college degree attainment in our example, we simply add an additional covariate, in this case allowing the covariate to have a time-varying effect, as follows:

$$SAT_i = \beta_0(t) + \beta_1(t)SEX_i + \beta_2(t)COLLEGE_i + \epsilon_i,$$

where SAT_i represents the career satisfaction score for individual i, SEX_i indicates individual i's sex, and $COLLEGE_i$ indicates whether individual i has a college degree. $\beta_0(t)$ is the intercept function, which now represents the estimated mean career satisfaction score as a continuous function across ages 25–65 for female adults with no college degree (i.e., where $SEX = 0$ and $COLLEGE = 0$), $\beta_1(t)$ is the coefficient function for *SEX*, representing the estimated difference in career satisfaction for male versus female adults across ages 25–65 controlling for college degree attainment, $\beta_2(t)$ is the coefficient function for college degree attainment holding sex constant, and the error term, ϵ_i, reflects individual i's deviation from their expected career satisfaction (i.e., the difference between their observed and expected career satisfaction for an adult of their specific age, sex, and college degree status). Thus, at each specific age, we can interpret the association between sex and career satisfaction holding college degree attainment constant. The variables needed to estimate this model include *CASEID*, *AGE*, *SAT*, *INT*, *SEX*, and *COLLEGE*.

To estimate this model, we specified a %TVEM macro statement in SAS.

```
%TVEM(
data = career_chapter2a,
dist = normal,
id = caseid,
time = age,
dv = sat,
tvary_effect = int sex college,
method = P-spline,
knots = 10 10 10);
```

The arguments are nearly identical to those in Model 2, with the following exceptions. We added the binary indicator of college degree attainment to the **tvary_effect** argument, which now includes three variables: *INT*, *SEX*, and *COLLEGE*. Three coefficient functions will be estimated: an intercept function and two slope functions for *SEX* and *COLLEGE*. Because we added a third variable with a time-varying effect, the **knots** statement now lists three values indicating the maximum number of knots to be considered for each coefficient function. We list 10 knots for each, and the P-spline algorithm automatically selects the optimal number of knots for all three coefficient functions.

Alternatively, one may choose to add a statistical control variable and specify that its coefficient has a time-invariant, as opposed to time-varying, effect. To do so, we simply add an additional covariate to Model 2, but in this case specify that its effect is time-invariant (i.e., the effect is constant across age), as follows:

$$SAT_i = \beta_0(t) + \beta_1(t) SEX_i + \beta_2 COLLEGE_i + \epsilon_i,$$

where β_2 is the parameter estimate representing the effect of college degree attainment. This is in contrast to the coefficient function, $\beta_2(t)$, as described above. To estimate this model, we specify a %TVEM macro statement in SAS.

```
%TVEM(
data = career_chapter2a,
dist = normal,
id = caseid,
time = age,
dv = sat,
tvary_effect = int sex,
method = P-spline,
knots = 10 10,
invar_effect = college);
```

In comparison to Model 2, this specification adds one new argument, **invar_effect**, which specifies the variable *COLLEGE*. Because only two coefficient functions are estimated, the intercept function and the coefficient for sex, only two values are required in the **knots** argument. A single coefficient is estimated for the effect of college degree attainment, and its effect is assumed to be constant across age.

The difference in interpretation when including statistical control variables with time-invariant versus time-varying effects is quite subtle, but we encourage researchers to work interpretations carefully to maintain precision. In both parameterizations for including college degree attainment as a statistical control variable, $\beta_1(t)$ reflects the age-varying association between sex, and career satisfaction is the coefficient function for *SEX* controlling for college degree attainment. The subtle difference can only be discerned when thinking very specifically about a point along the curve of $\beta_1(t)$. For example, suppose the coefficient for *sex* at age 30 is $\beta_1(30) = 4.5$. When specifying a time-varying effect for *COLLEGE*, we can interpret this quite precisely as "among adults who are 30 years old, male adults have a mean career satisfaction score that is 4.5 units higher than female adults, controlling for whether adults that age have a college degree." In other words, the effect of the statistical control is specific to that age. In contrast, when specifying a time-invariant effect for *COLLEGE*, we would interpret this a bit less precisely as "controlling for whether adults have a college degree, male adults who are age 30 have a mean career satisfaction score that is 4.5 units higher than female adults who are age 30." Again, the difference is quite subtle; we generally recommend that researchers specify the model both ways to determine whether it has any impact on the coefficient functions of interest (in this case, the effect of sex), and if not, opt for the more parsimonious model with a time-invariant effect of the statistical control variable. If it does have an impact on the coefficient functions of interest, we would suggest allowing the statistical control variable to have a time-varying effect as it more precisely maps onto the interpretation of the coefficient functions of interest.

2.3.4 *Model 4: Time-Varying Moderation*

Moderation analysis in TVEM often addresses some of the most interesting questions. Importantly, moderation effects themselves can be time-varying. Building on Model 3, we now add the interaction between sex and college degree attainment to the model with both main effects. The interaction term is specified to have a time-varying effect so that the age-varying sex difference can change with age differently for those with and without a college degree. We refer to this as *time-varying moderation*, where the effect of the moderator may vary across the age range. Note that we build on the version of Model 3 that specifies a time-varying effect for college degree attainment. This is important to maintain the hierarchical nature of the model; in other words, if the interaction term has a time-varying effect, both main effects for the variables that comprise the interaction term should have time-varying effects. To specify this moderation model, we simply add the variable that represents the product of *SEX* and *COLLEGE* and allow this term to have a time-varying effect, as follows:

$$SAT_i = \beta_0(t) + \beta_1(t)SEX_i + \beta_2(t)COLLEGE_i + \beta_3(t)SEX\_COLLEGE_i + \epsilon_i,$$

where SAT_i represents the career satisfaction score for individual *i*, SEX_i indicates individual *i*'s sex, $COLLEGE_i$ indicates whether individual *i* has a college degree, and $SEX\_COLLEGE_i$ indicates an individual's product between *SEX* and *COLLEGE*. $\beta_0(t)$ is the intercept function, which still represents the estimated mean career satisfaction score as a continuous function across ages 25–65 for female adults with no college degree (i.e., where $SEX = 0$ and $COLLEGE = 0$), $\beta_1(t)$ is the coefficient function for the main effect of *SEX*, representing the estimated difference in career satisfaction for male compared to female adults across ages 25–65 among adults with no college degree. $\beta_2(t)$ is the coefficient function for the main effect of college degree attainment, representing the estimated increase (or decrease) in career satisfaction for those with a college degree compared to those without a college degree across ages 25–65 among female adults. $\beta_3(t)$ is the coefficient function for the interaction between sex and college degree attainment, representing the age-varying difference in the age-varying sex gap in career satisfaction among those with a college degree compared to those without a college degree. The error term, ϵ_i, reflects individual *i*'s deviation from their expected career satisfaction (i.e., the difference between their observed and expected career satisfaction for an adult of their specific age, sex, and college degree status).

The coefficient function for the interaction term, $\beta_3(t)$, allows us to conduct nuanced hypothesis testing of college degree attainment as a moderator of the association between sex and career satisfaction. Ages at which the confidence interval of the interaction term's coefficient does not include the value zero indicate that college degree attainment operates as a moderator of the sex difference in career satisfaction. In other words, at each specific age, we can examine the statistical significance of and interpret the association between sex and career satisfaction for those with a college degree and for those without a college degree. The same set of variables used in Model 3 is needed to estimate this model: *CASEID*, *AGE*, *SAT*, *INT*, *SEX*, and *COLLEGE*.

To estimate this time-varying moderation model, we specified a %TVEM macro statement in SAS.

```
%TVEM(
data = career_chapter2a,
dist = normal,
id = caseid,
time = age,
dv = sat,
tvary_effect = int sex college sex_college,
method = P-spline,
knots = 10 10 10 10);
```

The arguments are nearly identical to those in Model 3, with the following exceptions. We added the binary product term for sex by college degree attainment to the **tvary_effect** argument, which now includes four variables: *INT*, *SEX*, *COLLEGE*, and *SEX_COLLEGE*. Four coefficient functions will be estimated: an intercept function, two slope functions for the main effects of *SEX* and *COLLEGE*, and a slope function for the interaction term. Because we added a fourth variable with a time-varying effect, the **knots** statement now lists four values indicating the number of knots for each coefficient function. We list 10 knots for each of the 3 coefficient functions to allow the model to estimate nuanced coefficient functions; the P-spline algorithm automatically controls the amount of change that should be accommodated at each knot to avoid overfitting the curves to the data. Again, in our experience curves estimated using P-spline with 10 knots appear essentially the same as those with 5 knots specified; however, there is essentially no cost to specifying a larger number of knots.

As with classic multiple linear regression, significant interaction terms require careful interpretation. For example, if our analysis ignored age and the coefficient for *SEX_COLLEGE* were statistically significant, we most likely would present the simple slopes to aid interpretation. That is, we would present the effect of sex (the simple slope of sex) for those with a college degree and also present the effect of sex for those without a college degree. Similarly, in TVEM the most effective way to unpack coefficient functions for interaction terms is to examine estimated coefficient functions at different levels of a moderating variable; in this case, to examine the coefficient function for sex for those with and without a college degree. We encourage researchers who wish to interpret time-varying moderation effects to (1) present the coefficient function for the interaction term (in our example, $\beta_3(t)$), (2) describe the specific time/age ranges at which the moderation effect is significant, and (3) plot simple slope coefficient functions for different levels of the moderator. These simple slope functions can be obtained in two ways in TVEM. One can combine the values of the coefficient functions from the main effects and interaction term, for example, in a spreadsheet program like Excel. This approach is most straightforward for categorical moderators, but simple slope functions in TVEM can be obtained similarly for continuous moderators, for example, by calculating the slope functions at 1 SD above and 1 SD below the mean on the moderator. An example involving a categorical moderator is presented in Chap. 3. The companion website for this book (https://prevention.psu.edu/books/tvem/) presents further detail on how to use TVEM output to manually create tailored plots using Excel. Alternatively, TVEM has an optional **domain** argument that allows simple slope functions to be automatically calculated and plotted across levels of a categorical moderator. This useful approach is demonstrated below.

2.4 Empirical Example: Age-Varying Association Between Closeness to Mother and Depressive Symptoms

In this section, we demonstrate how to develop a time-varying effect model to predict depressive symptoms across adolescence and young adulthood from closeness to mother and the moderating role of participant's sex. Specifically, we pose the following research questions:

Research Question 1: What is the mean level of depressive symptoms across age in a national sample of individuals followed from adolescence through young adulthood?

Research Question 2: What is the age-varying association between maternal closeness during adolescence and depressive symptoms prospectively through young adulthood?

Research Question 3: Does This age-varying association differ between female and male individuals?

To address these research questions, we will examine public-use data from the National Longitudinal Study of Adolescent to Adult Health (Add Health), a longitudinal panel study of individuals in the United States that began with Wave 1 in 1994–1995, when adolescents were in Grades 7–12. We examine data from the first four waves of Add Health, where Wave 2 was conducted in 1996, Wave 3 in 2001–2002, and Wave 4 in 2008–2009. This can be thought of as an accelerated longitudinal design, as individuals at different ages were recruited and followed up at subsequent time points to more efficiently collect data across a larger age range. Thus, although each participant only provided data at a maximum of four measurement occasions, when combining across participants and occasions, excellent coverage is achieved across ages 13–32 years. In this study, raw age was used as our "time" variable thus observations were aligned in terms of time relative to birth (i.e., time 0 represents the time of birth).

Given that Add Health was designed to produce results that could be interpreted as nationally representative and our interest in describing age-varying associations, we did not model all available data from the original Wave 1 sample of 6504 adolescents. Rather, we used the longitudinal data with responses from Waves 1–4 merged together and only included individuals who had a sample weight at the final time point (Wave 4). This reduced our analysis sample to $n = 3342$ individuals who continued to participate through Wave 4 but allowed us to avoid the potential serious limitation of having the sample composition change with age. This approach does not necessarily address all missing data across waves (e.g., an individual still participating at Wave 4 may have missed taking the Wave 2 assessment or may have chosen not to respond to all variables of interest at one wave), but by eliminating important and sizeable attrition effects, our findings could more plausibly be interpreted as age trends in the associations. The Add Health study released sample weights specifically designed for longitudinal modeling across Waves 1–4; all models examined here included this sample weight and adjusted for the nested structure inherent in repeated-measures data.

In this example, depressive symptoms are a repeatedly assessed continuous scale score, and closeness to mother and participant's sex are assessed with single items at Wave 1, during adolescence. Although these data naturally lend themselves to addressing questions such as *"How is adolescent closeness to mother related to individual growth trajectories in depressive symptoms over time?"* (which could be addressed using a linear growth curve model), in this study our interest is in addressing questions such as *"How does the association between adolescent closeness to mother and current depressive symptoms vary as a flexible function of age?"* A more detailed discussion of the differences between linear growth curve modeling and TVEM is presented in Chap. 7. We note that if closeness to mother had been assessed at every time point, the value of this covariate could be time-varying within each individual. The model specification would be identical, and only the interpretation would change. Specifically, instead of addressing the question, *"How does the association between* ***adolescent*** *closeness to mother and current depressive symptoms vary as a flexible function of age?"* the analysis would address the question, *"How does the association between* ***current*** *closeness to mother and current depressive symptoms vary as a flexible function of age?"*

The outcome we wish to model is the level of depressive symptoms, measured with a common instrument at each of the four waves. This variable was calculated as the mean across responses to nine questions assessing recent (past 2 weeks in Waves 1 and 2, past week in Waves 3 and 4) symptoms, each scored 0, 1, 2, or 3. Response options were 0 = never or rarely, 1 = sometimes, 2 = a lot of the time, and

Table 2.2 Descriptive statistics for continuous variables to be used in analysis ($n = 3342$)

Variable		Effective N	Weighted mean	Standard deviation
Age	Wave 1	3340	15.50	1.58
	Wave 2	3341	16.41	1.59
	Wave 3	3341	21.87	1.61
	Wave 4	3341	28.37	1.61
Closeness to mother at Wave 1		3314	4.53	0.81
Depressive symptoms	Wave 1	3337	0.62	0.46
	Wave 2	3339	0.63	0.47
	Wave 3	3341	0.51	0.45
	Wave 4	3341	0.57	0.45

3 = most of the time or all of the time. Individual items were reverse-coded as necessary so that higher numbers correspond to more severe symptoms. The symptoms were: bothered by things; had the blues; just as good as other people (reversed); trouble keeping mind focused; felt depressed; too tired to do things; enjoyed life (reversed); felt sad; and felt people dislike you.

The analytic sample is 50.3% (weighted) male. Weighted descriptive statistics for continuous variables to be used to address the current research questions are shown in Table 2.2. We will return to this empirical example throughout the remainder of this chapter to demonstrate the concepts presented next, including data considerations, model specification and estimation, and model interpretation.

Due to extreme sparseness of observations at ages younger than 13 and older than 32 years, we restricted our analysis to 13,205 (of 13,368 total) assessments across the four waves when participants were across ages 13–32. Thus, all weighted coefficient functions are estimated and presented for the age range of 13–32 years. Before specifying our first TVEM, we examined the distributional properties of the outcome, which ranged from 0–3 with an overall mean score on depressive symptoms of 0.59. The distribution had positive skew (skewness = 1.19, indicating a right skew compared to a normal distribution of skewness = 0) and high kurtosis (kurtosis = 1.62, indicating heavier tails compared to a normal distribution of kurtosis = 0) thus we applied a square-root transformation which resulted in a distribution that was much better approximated by a normal distribution (skewness = −0.14, kurtosis = −0.02, min = 0, max = 1.73).

2.4.1 Research Question 1: What is the Mean Level of Depressive Symptoms Across Age in a National Sample of Individuals Followed From Adolescence Through Young Adulthood?

An intercept-only model was used to estimate the mean depressive symptom score across age. The model specified here is

$$DEP_i = \beta_0(t) + \epsilon_i,$$

where DEP_i indicates individual i's scale score for depressive symptoms (in this case, the square-root of their mean across 9 depressive symptoms), and $\beta_0(t)$ is the coefficient function (i.e., intercept function) for the estimated mean depressive symptom score across continuous age. To estimate this model, we specified a %WeightedTVEM macro statement in SAS.

```
%WeightedTVEM(
data = chap2.add_long,
dist = normal,
cluster = aid,
time = age,
dv = sq_dep,
tvary_effect = int,
knots = 4,
weight = gswgt4);
```

The **data** statement is the name of our analysis dataset. The **cluster** statement refers to our participant ID variable; because this study used a longitudinal panel design with four waves, individuals can have up to four rows in our vertical dataset. The **cluster** statement ensures that the estimate of standard errors takes into account the nested data structure inherent in repeated-measures data. **Time** refers to the variable to use on the x-axis, which in this case is age (which ranges in the dataset from 13 to 32 years). **DV** is the argument for our outcome variable, in this case, the square-root of the depressive symptoms score, denoted as *SQ_DEP*. The outcome is continuous thus we specify a "normal" distribution in the **dist** argument. Because this simple model evaluates only the estimated mean of the dependent variable (*SQ_DEP*) across age, our **tvary_effect** includes only the intercept. We have already created a variable in our dataset (called *INT*), which is equal to 1 for all rows of data.

The **knots** statement refers to the number of splitting points we are specifying for any time-varying effects being estimated, with a higher number corresponding to a more complex coefficient function. The **weight** argument lists the variable containing the sample weights (*GSWGT4*). Because we are analyzing weighted data, B-spline estimation is used to estimate the coefficient function, and we must perform model selection (i.e., choose the optimal number of knots) manually. The intercept-only model only estimates a single coefficient function; we compared models with 1 through 5 knots (see Table 2.3; selected number of knots bolded for emphasis).

We selected 4 knots for our final model (i.e., Model 2), as it had the lowest AIC and BIC values thus suggesting an optimal balance between fit and parsimony. The model with four knots corresponds to a fairly complex, nonlinear function. We show the estimated intercept coefficient function $\beta_0(t)$ and its corresponding 95% confidence interval in Fig. 2.1. At each age, the coefficient reflects the estimated mean

Table 2.3 Model fit information for selecting the optimal number of knots for the intercept function

Model #	# Knots for *INT*	AIC	BIC
1	5	7606.71	7674.10
2	**4**	**7606.25**	**7666.16**
3	3	7614.35	7666.76
4	2	7628.16	7673.09
5	1	7629.38	7666.82

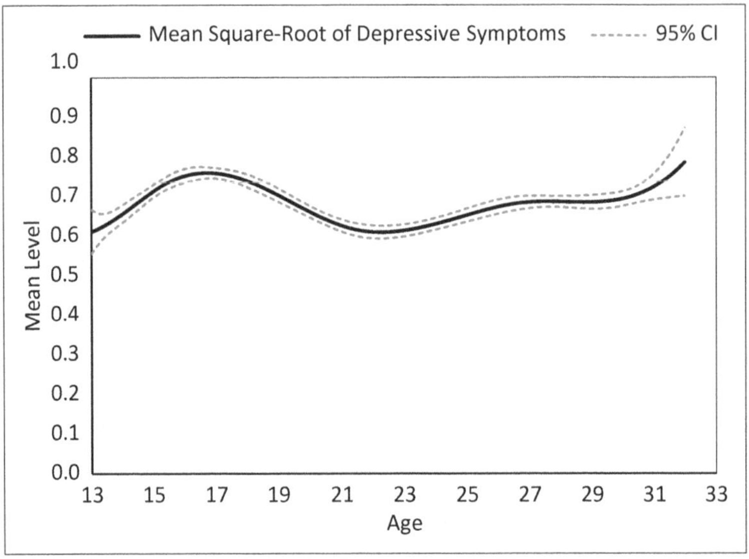

Fig. 2.1 Mean square-root of depressive symptoms across ages 13–32 years

square-root of depressive symptoms. Notice the nuanced curve shape, which would be impossible to capture with a simpler parametric function, such as linear or quadratic.

When a model is estimated using the macro, a data file also is automatically created that contains values from the estimated coefficient function(s). By default, these estimates are stored in the file **tvem_plot_data**. This file contains the data SAS used to create the figures; thus, researchers may access this dataset directly if they wish to recreate figures in the software of their choice. The **tvem_plot_data** file, by default, contains 100 records, with the first row corresponding to the lowest time plotted (in this case, age 13 years) and the last row corresponding to the highest time (in this case, age 32 years). The remaining 98 rows are equally spaced between the lowest and highest time and contain values of the coefficient function and corresponding confidence limits across the 100 equally spaced intervals. In our example, the first row of the dataset corresponds to age 13, with an estimated coefficient of 0.611 (i.e., the expected square-root of depressive symptoms score is 0.611 at age 13), an estimated standard error of 0.028, and 95% confidence interval of [0.555–0.666]. Our last row of the dataset (age 32) has an estimated coefficient of 0.786, standard error of 0.044, and 95% confidence interval of [0.700–0.872]. The companion website (https://prevention.psu.edu/books/tvem/) includes a demonstration for creating publication-ready figures in Excel using this file. Note that the default number of records in the **tvem_plot_data** file can be changed using the optional **plot_scale** argument to achieve a more or less dense set of points from which to plot curves.

Referring to Fig. 2.1, we see that the lowest mean depressive symptoms were observed at age 13 and the highest was observed at age 32, but the shape of the curve across age was far from linear. Rather, we see a relatively steep increase with age between ages 13 and 16 years, peaking at just over age 16, and then decreasing with age into young adulthood. After about age 23, we observe a slow but consistent increase with age in depressive symptoms, with the steepest increase with age observed between ages 30 and 32 years. At all ages, the confidence interval is narrow, reflecting the high level of confidence in our estimates across the entire age range. The slight flare in the width of confidence intervals at the endpoints (ages 13, 32) is typical for TVEM, as spline-based regression procedures borrow information from nearby times to estimate a point on the curve; because there is no information at ages below 13 or above 32, we tend to see confidence intervals widen close to the endpoints.

2.4.2 Research Question 2: What is the Age-Varying Association Between Maternal Closeness During Adolescence and Depressive Symptoms Prospectively Through Young Adulthood?

A main-effects TVEM was used to estimate the mean depressive symptom score as a function of closeness to mother, across age. The model specified here is

$$DEP_i = \beta_0(t) + \beta_1(t)CLOSMOM1_i + \epsilon_i,$$

where depression symptoms (DEP_i) indicate the square-root of individual i's scale score and $CLOSMOM1_i$ represents individual i's self-reported closeness to their mother at Wave 1. $\beta_0(t)$ is the intercept function representing expected mean depressive symptoms across age when closeness to mother equals zero, and $\beta_1(t)$ is the coefficient function representing the expected change on mean (square-root) depressive symptoms associated with a one-unit increase in closeness to mother, across age. To estimate this model, we specified a %WeightedTVEM macro statement in SAS.

```
%WeightedTVEM(
data = chap2.add_chapter2,
dist = normal,
cluster = aid,
time = age,
dv = sq_dep,
tvary_effect = int closmom1,
knots = 4 1,
weight = gswgt4);
```

This model is a modified version of the intercept-only TVEM specified above. As this regression model estimates the association between closeness to mother at Wave 1 (*CLOSMOM1*) and our dependent variable (square-root of depressive symptoms, *SQ_DEP*) across age, our **tvary_effect** argument includes an intercept and a coefficient for closeness to mother. Note that both the intercept and slope coefficients are specified to be time-varying, indicating that both mean depressive symptoms and the association between closeness to mother and depressive symptoms can vary with age. We now have to specify two values in the **knots** argument: one for the coefficient function for *INT* and another for the coefficient function for *CLOSMOM1*. As in the intercept-only model above, model selection must be performed manually to select the number of knots—keeping in mind that the optimal number of knots need not be the same for all coefficient functions.

To conduct model selection in TVEM involving two coefficient functions, we recommend setting the number of knots for the intercept to a larger number, say 5, and varying the number of knots specified for the slope function. (In our experience, a maximum of 5 knots is nearly always sufficient; more than 5 knots need only be considered if one has reason to expect that systematic change over time may be quite complex.) Based on the minimum AIC and/or BIC, one can first select the number of knots for the slope function and then hold that number constant when considering the selection of other numbers of knots. In our example, we initially held the number of knots for the intercept function to be 5 and compared models with 1 through 5 knots on the slope function (i.e., the coefficient for *CLOSMOM1*; see fit statistics for Models 1 through 5 in Table 2.4). Among these, the model with 1 knot was selected based on the lower BIC (Model 5: BIC=7376.07) and extremely minor difference in AIC when comparing Model 4 (AIC=7271.30) and Model 5 (AIC=7271.35). In cases where the choice of a number of knots is not clear, one may wish to inspect the estimated coefficient functions from competing models; in our example, differences between the coefficient function for *CLOSMOM1* in Models 4 and 5 were not meaningful. We then set the number of knots for the slope function to 1, then compared models with 1 through 5 knots for the intercept function (see fit statistics for Models 5 through 9 in Table 2.4). Among these, we selected Model 6, with 4 knots for the intercept function and 1 knot for the slope

Table 2.4 Model fit information for selecting the optimal number of knots for the intercept and slope coefficient functions

Model #	# Knots for *INT*	# Knots for *CLOSMOM1*	AIC	BIC
1	5	5	7269.47	7404.11
2	5	4	7273.34	7400.51
3	5	3	7271.79	7391.47
4	5	2	7271.30	7383.51
5	5	1	7271.35	7376.07
6	**4**	**1**	**7271.04**	**7368.28**
7	3	1	7284.15	7373.91
8	2	1	7286.33	7368.62
9	1	1	7299.42	7374.22

function, as our final model (see Table 2.4; selected number of knots bolded for emphasis).

In Fig. 2.2 we show the estimated coefficient functions, $\beta_0(t)$ and $\beta_1(t)$, and their corresponding 95% confidence intervals. The intercept function (Fig. 2.2a) is not terribly meaningful, as it represents the expected depressive symptoms score for individuals with a 0 on closeness to mother. As in classic multiple linear regression, covariates may be centered in any way desired to facilitate interpretation. For example, closeness to mother could be centered so that 0 represents the mean score in the sample; in this case, the intercept function is interpreted as the expected depressive symptoms across age for individuals with mean closeness to mother at Wave 1.

Coefficient functions corresponding to covariates in the model can be complex to interpret, as researchers are used to interpreting a single-number summary of an association. We recommend first examining broad features of the coefficient function and then focusing on key details. For example, one could examine features of a function to address questions such as the following:

- *Are there ages at which the association is significantly different from 0? If so, at what ages?*
- *During any ages at which the coefficient is significant, is the association positive or negative?*
- *At what age is the strength of association the strongest? What is the effect size at that age and its interpretation? At what age is the strength of association the weakest?*
- *At what ages is the change in the strength of association the most pronounced?*

The coefficient function for closeness to mother (Fig. 2.2b) is negative at all ages, and the 95% confidence bands do not include 0 between ages 13 and 31 years. Because the confidence bands above age 31 cross the horizontal line where the

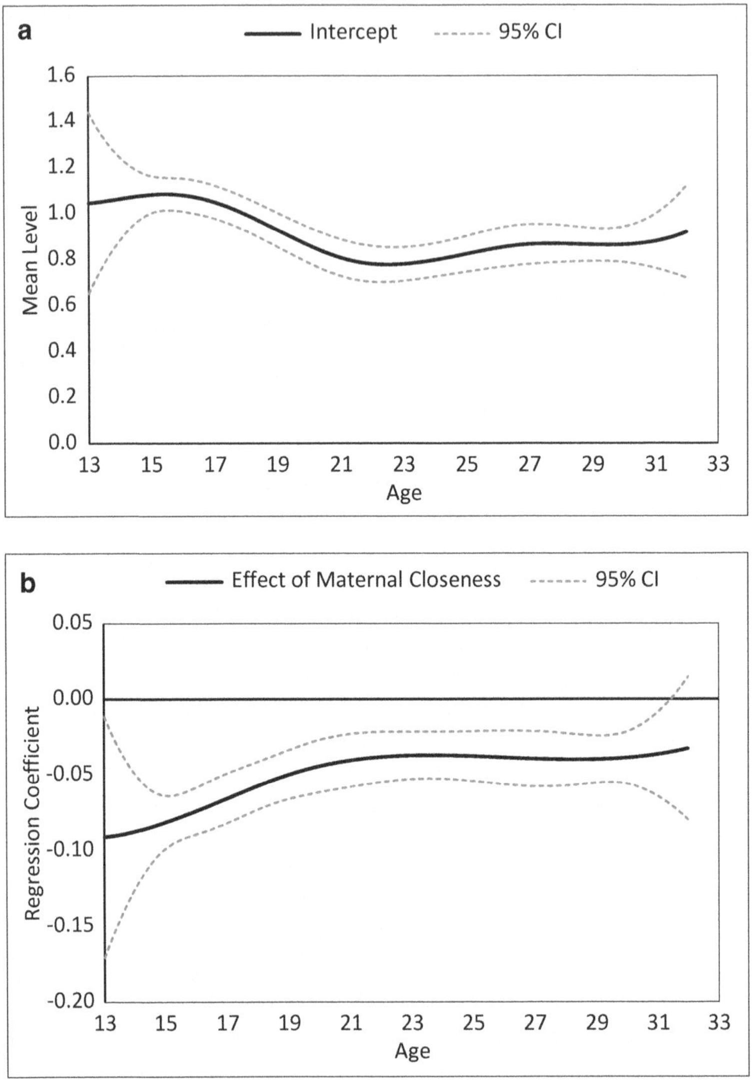

Fig. 2.2 Coefficient functions from main effect model predicting depressive symptoms across ages 13–32 years. (**a**) Intercept function, reflecting estimated mean depressive symptoms at maternal closeness of 0. (**b**) Slope function, reflecting the estimated difference in depressive symptoms associated with a one-unit increase in maternal closeness

coefficient estimate is 0, the association is not statistically significant at that age. The significant, negative association from ages 13 to 31 indicates that individuals who report greater closeness to mother report significantly fewer depressive symptoms, on average. This association is strongest in early adolescence, specifically around ages 13–15 years. At age 13, the estimated association is approximately −0.9, indicating that for every one-unit increase on closeness with mother (on a 5-point scale), the outcome is expected to be 0.9 units lower. As the outcome in our models was transformed to reflect the square-root of the depressive symptoms score, by squaring it we can expect the mean depressive score to be about 0.8 points lower on the original scale of 0–3 for every one-unit increase on closeness to mother. In sum, this figure shows that closeness to mother may be most protective during early adolescence, with the effect weakening with age throughout adolescence, then maintaining a small but significant association throughout ages 20–31. We note that for time-varying covariates it often is valuable to estimate an intercept-only TVEM with the covariate specified as the outcome; this can provide valuable descriptive information about the time-varying mean on the covariate. However, in this example recall that closeness to mother was assessed at Wave 1 only and specified as a time-invariant covariate with a time-varying effect.

2.4.3 Research Question 3: Does This Age-Varying Association Differ Between Female and Male Individuals?

Examining differences between male and female individuals in the age-varying association between closeness to mother and depressive symptoms is a moderation question. Thus, we specify a time-varying effect model that includes a main effect for closeness to mother, a main effect for sex, and their interaction. Because all coefficients are estimated as a function of continuous age, we can consider this an examination of age-varying moderation. The model specified here is

$$DEP_i = \beta_0(t) + \beta_1(t)CLOSMOM1_i + \beta_2(t)MALE_i + \beta_3(t)M\_CLOSMOM_i + \epsilon_i,$$

where depression symptoms (DEP_i) indicate individual i's scale score, $CLOSMOM1_i$ represents individual i's self-reported closeness to their mother at Wave 1, $MALE_i$ represents individual i's self-reported sex (coded 0 = female, 1 = male), and $M\_CLOSMOM_i$ represents individual i's product of sex and closeness to mother. Four coefficient functions are estimated. $\beta_0(t)$ is the intercept function representing expected mean depressive symptoms across age for female individuals with closeness to mother equal to zero, $\beta_1(t)$ is the coefficient function representing the main effect of closeness to mother across age, $\beta_2(t)$ is the coefficient function representing the main effect of being male across age, and $\beta_3(t)$ is the coefficient function representing the interaction of closeness to mother and sex, across age. It is this coefficient function that enables the age-varying statistical test of sex differences in the closeness to mother-depressive symptoms association. To estimate this model, we specified a %WeightedTVEM macro statement in SAS.

```
%WeightedTVEM(
data = chap2.add_chapter2,
dist = normal,
cluster = aid,
time = age,
dv = sq_dep,
tvary_effect = int closmom1 male m_closmom,
knots = 4 1 1 1,
weight = gswgt4);
```

This model is a modified version of the main-effect TVEM specified above. Our **tvary_effect** now specifies an intercept, main effects for closeness to mother and for sex, and an interaction term. Note that all coefficients are specified to be time-varying; we recommend that if the interaction term has a time-varying effect, so should the main effects of variables that comprise the interaction term. We now have to specify four values in the **knots** argument, the first for the coefficient function for *INT*, the second and third for the main effects of *CLOSMOM1* and *MALE*, respectively, and the fourth for the moderation effect, *M_CLOSMOM*. Model selection must be performed to select each number of knots, as weighted TVEM requires that we use B-spline estimation. It is important to keep in mind that the suggested number of knots need not be the same for all coefficient functions. We walk the reader through this process of selecting the number of knots below, as well as in several empirical examples in Chap. 3.

Relying on the AIC and BIC, we first selected the number of knots for the interaction term; then selected the number of knots for the coefficient functions for sex and closeness to mother, respectively; and finally selected the number of knots for the intercept function. Considering a maximum of 5 knots per function, this model selection procedure required us to compare 17 models (see Table 2.5). In our example, we held the number of knots for the first three functions to be 5 and compared models with 1 through 5 knots on the coefficient function for the interaction term (Models 1–5 in Table 2.5) and selected 1 knot for this function. Following a similar procedure, we compared Models 5–9 and selected 1 knot for the coefficient function for sex. Next, we compared Models 9–13 and selected 1 knot for the coefficient function for closeness to mother. Finally, we compared Models 13–17 to select the number of knots for the intercept function. Table 2.5 shows model fit information for all candidate models; selected number of knots bolded for emphasis. The AIC indicated that the 4-knot model was optimal, whereas the BIC indicated that the 2-knot model was best. As the BIC tends to favor parsimony more than the AIC, we opted to select Model 16 as our final model, with 2 knots in the intercept function and 1 knot in each of the slope functions. Importantly, we visually inspected the interaction coefficient function for Models 14 and 16, and the results were nearly identical—thus, no important information was lost by choosing the more parsimonious model in this case. Interestingly, if one scans the AIC for all models considered here, Model 9 has the lowest AIC overall (AIC=7048.75), although the AIC for Model 14 was not meaningfully higher (AIC=7048.96). As with any statistical

Table 2.5 Model fit information for selecting the optimal number of knots for the intercept and slope functions

Model #	# Knots for *INT*	# Knots for *CLOSMOM1*	# Knots for *MALE*	# Knots for *M_CLOSMOM*	AIC	BIC
1	5	5	5	5	7062.03	7331.31
2	5	5	5	4	7060.79	7322.60
3	5	5	5	3	7060.14	7314.46
4	5	5	5	2	7058.37	7305.21
5	5	5	5	1	7056.30	7295.64
6	5	5	4	1	7054.90	7286.78
7	5	5	3	1	7052.75	7276.98
8	5	5	2	1	7051.78	7268.71
9	5	5	1	1	7048.75	7258.19
10	5	4	1	1	7054.89	7256.85
11	5	3	1	1	7052.07	7246.55
12	5	2	1	1	7052.55	7239.55
13	5	1	1	1	7049.78	7229.30
14	4	1	1	1	7048.96	7221.00
15	3	1	1	1	7062.40	7226.97
16	**2**	**1**	**1**	**1**	**7060.20**	**7217.28**
17	1	1	1	1	7082.42	7232.02

model, researchers may rely on multiple information criteria for model selection, but must be aware that they often do not agree on the optimal balance between fit and parsimony. This is due to the different levels of priority given to the penalization term (We refer the interested reader to Dziak, Coffman, Lanza, Li, & Jermiin, 2020, for a thorough comparison of information criteria for conducting model selection.).

We show the estimated coefficient function for the interaction term, $\beta_3(t)$, and its corresponding 95% confidence interval in Fig. 2.3. As in classic multiple linear regression, an interaction term that is statistically different from 0 indicates moderation. Although technically the confidence interval at age 13 does not include 0, the interval is quite wide here. Additionally, this very small region of significance was not significant when a different number of knots was specified. Therefore, we will not interpret this age period. Rather, we focus on the age range of 22–26 years, where there is a significant positive effect of the interaction term. In other words, we do detect significant moderation by sex in the association between closeness to mother and depressive symptoms, but only during this age period in young adulthood.

Interpreting interaction terms in multiple regression analysis always requires careful attention. It is even more challenging in the context of TVEM, where a moderation effect is time-varying. Not shown here is the intercept function or the main effect functions. The easiest way to address our specific research question on moderation (i.e., to interpret the significant moderation effect identified in this model) is to add a **domain** argument in the TVEM syntax as follows.

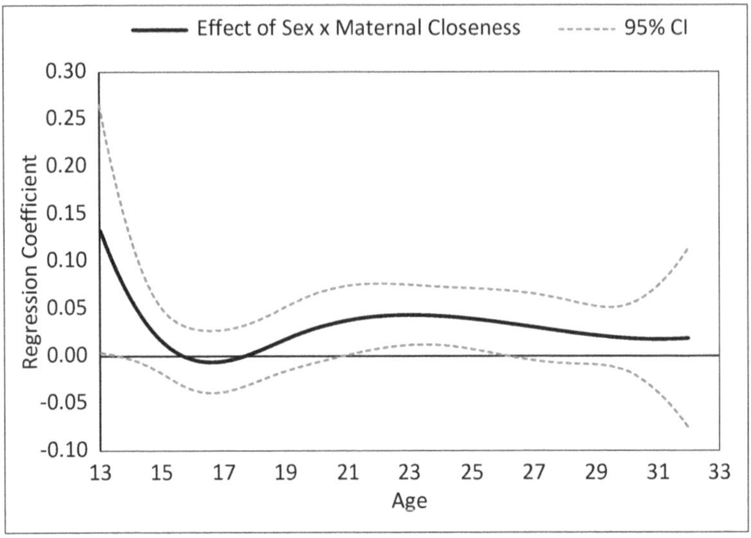

Fig. 2.3 Coefficient function for term representing the interaction between sex and maternal closeness in predicting depressive symptoms across ages 13–32 years

```
%WeightedTVEM(
data = chap2.add_chapter2,
dist = normal,
cluster = aid,
time = age,
dv = sq_dep,
tvary_effect = int closmom1,
knots = 2 1,
weight = gswgt4,
domain = male,
which = 1);
```

In this syntax, we specify in the **tvary_effect** argument only the terms for the intercept and closeness to mother (but remove terms for sex and the interaction). We then add the **domain** argument, indicating that *MALE* is the variable by which we want to examine the simple slope function for closeness with mother. Finally, we add the **which** argument and specify the value of 1; this will produce the desired simple slope function for male individuals (where *MALE* = 1). This produces the age-varying effect of closeness to mother on depressive symptoms for male individuals, using an appropriately weighted analysis; this coefficient function appears in Fig. 2.4a. Finally, in the **which** argument we replace 1 with 0 to produce the same age-varying effect of closeness to mother on depressive symptoms and rerun the model, this time obtaining the coefficient function for closeness to mother for female individuals; this coefficient function is shown in Fig. 2.4b. To facilitate

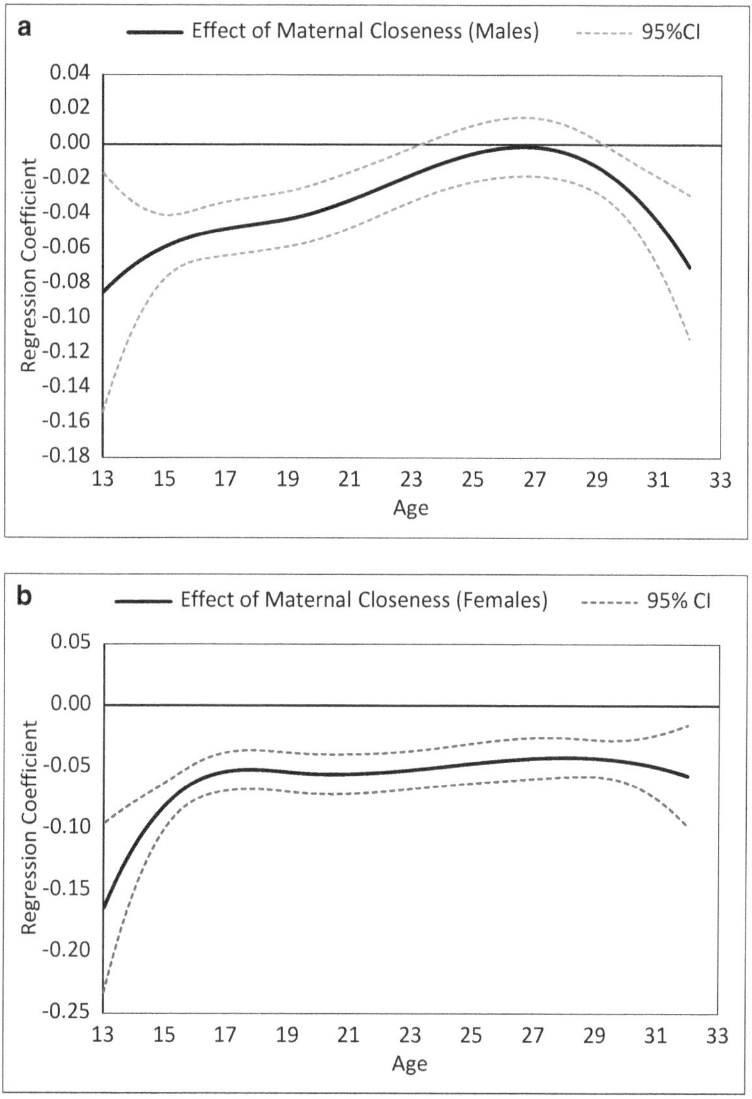

Fig. 2.4 Simple slopes showing the association between maternal closeness and depressive symptoms for (**a**) males and (**b**) females

male-female comparison, one may wish to reproduce Fig. 2.4a, b on the same graph; however, Fig. 2.3 should be relied upon to test for ages at which significant moderation is detected.

To interpret Fig. 2.4a, b, it is helpful to recall the age range at which significant moderation was detected (approximately ages 22–26, as shown in Fig. 2.3). The coefficient function for male is significant and negative at ages 13–23 years, and then at ages 29–32 years, but the association between closeness to mother and depressive symptoms was not significant between ages 23 and 29. In other words, for male individuals, closeness to mother at Wave 1 appears to potentially protect against depressive symptoms throughout adolescence and some periods of young adulthood, but not during the mid-20s. We also note that for male individuals, the strongest association was among those age 13 years, with a coefficient of about −0.08.

Among female adolescents, closeness to mother appears to have the strongest protective effect at age 13 as well, but the association is twice as strong as for male individuals, with a coefficient of about −0.16. Remember that the interaction term at age 13 had a wide confidence interval, so we must interpret this sex difference with caution. This potentially protective effect among female individuals weakens with age rapidly during adolescence, to about −0.05 by age 18, and then maintains a remarkably stable strength of association from ages 18–32 years. Recall that male and female individuals were statistically different in this association between ages 22 and 26 years. Taken together, these results show that closeness to mother at Wave 1 may be protective for both male and female adolescents against depressive symptoms, but this association is stronger among female adults during their early 20s and disappears for male adults in their mid-20s. Closeness to mother at Wave 1 however appears to be potentially protective for both male and female adults again toward the end of the age range (e.g., ages 28–32 years).

2.4.4 Sample Results Section

Sample Results Section: Maternal Closeness

Research Question 1. Model selection for the intercept-only model indicated that 4 knots was optimal. The estimated level of depressive symptoms across ages 13–32 years is presented in Fig. 2.1. Mean (square-root) depressive symptoms increased with age, from a minimum level of 0.61 (95% confidence interval = 0.56–0.67) at age 13 to a maximum level of 0.79 at age 32 (95% confidence interval = 0.70–0.87). The shape of change across age was not linear, but instead featured a steep increase across ages 13–16, peaking at just over age 16, and then decreasing with age into young adulthood. Mean depressive symptoms increased gradually with age after about age 23, with a sharper rise between ages 30–32.

Research Question 2. Maternal closeness was added as a predictor; model selection indicated that the optimal model had 4 knots for the intercept function and 2 knots for the coefficient function for maternal closeness. The association between maternal closeness during adolescence and depressive symptoms prospectively was statistically significant at every age across the age range (see Fig. 2.2b). The coefficient for maternal closeness is negative at all ages, indicating that adolescents who reported greater maternal closeness reported significantly fewer depressive symptoms, on average, across all ages.

The association between maternal closeness and depressive symptoms is strongest in early adolescence, specifically around ages 13–15 years. At age

13, the estimated association is approximately -0.9, indicating that for every one-unit increase on maternal closeness (on a 5-point scale), the outcome is expected to be 0.9 units lower. As this is the square-root of the mean depressive symptoms score, by squaring it we can expect the mean depressive score to be about .8 lower on the original metric (a scale of 0–3). In sum, this figure shows that maternal closeness may be most protective during early adolescence, with the association weakening with age throughout adolescence, then maintaining a small but significant protective effect throughout ages 20–31.

Research Question 3. Next, we examined sex differences in the age-varying association between maternal closeness and depressive symptoms. Model selection, which involved choosing the optimal number of knots for the intercept function and the coefficient functions for maternal closeness, sex, and their interaction, suggested 2, 1, 1, and 1 knots, respectively. Figure 2.3 shows the coefficient function for the interaction term, indicating statistically significant moderation between ages 22 and 26 years but not at ages below about 22 or over 26 years. To facilitate interpretation of this significant interaction coefficient function, we calculated the simple slope functions (i.e., the estimated association between maternal closeness and depressive symptoms across age for female and male individuals).

Among male individuals (Fig. 2.4a), the coefficient for maternal closeness is statistically significant and negative at ages 13–23 years and at ages 29–32 years, such that higher reported maternal closeness is associated with lower mean depressive symptoms. There was a noticeable absence of association between ages 23 and 29 years, suggesting that maternal closeness during adolescence may not be protective of male young adults. The strongest association, indicating potential protection, among male individuals was at age 13 years, with a coefficient of −0.08. Similar to male individuals, among female individuals (Fig. 2.4b), maternal closeness appeared to have the strongest association with depressive symptoms at age 13 years. However, this potentially protective effect was twice as strong for female individuals, with an age 13 coefficient of −0.16. The association among female individuals weakened with age rapidly during adolescence, to about -0.05 by age 18, and then maintained a remarkably stable strength of association from ages 18 to 32 years.

Recall that male and female adults were statistically different in this association between ages 22 and 26 years. Taken together, these results show that closeness to mom at Wave 1 may be protective against depressive symptoms for both male and female adolescents, but this association has more strength among female individuals during their early 20s and even disappears for male adults in their mid-20s. Closeness to mom at Wave 1 however again appears to be protective for both male and female adults toward the end of the age range (e.g., ages 28–32 years).

References

Dziak, J. J., Coffman, D. L., Lanza, S. T., Li, R., & Jermiin, L. S. (2020). Sensitivity and specificity of information criteria. *Briefings in Bioinformatics, 21*(2), 553–565.

Dziak, J. J., Li, R., & Wagner, A. (2017). *Weighted TVEM SAS macro users' guide (Version 2.6).* The Methodology Center, Penn State.

Eilers, P. H., & Marx, B. D. (1996). Flexible smoothing with B-splines and penalties. *Statistical Science, 11*, 89–102.

Li, R., Dziak, J. J., Tan, X., Huang, L., Wagner, A. T., & Yang, J. (2017). TVEM *(time-varying effect modeling) SAS macro users' guide, v. 3.1.1.* The Methodology Center, Penn State.

Liang, K.-Y., & Zeger, S. L. J. (1986). Longitudinal data analysis using generalized linear models. *Biometrika, 73*(1), 13–22.

Chapter 3
Generalized Time-Varying Effect Models for Binary and Count Outcomes

In addition to its application for modeling continuous outcomes, the time-varying effect model can be used to estimate time-varying prevalence and odds ratios for binary outcomes, such as the age-varying prevalence of cardiac arrests in the past year in a nationally representative sample of adults or the age-varying association between level of perceived stress and odds of having a cardiac arrest. Using Poisson time-varying effect modeling (TVEM), one can model count outcomes across time or the time-varying association between covariates and a count outcome across time. For example, TVEM could estimate the mean number of servings of fruits and vegetables an individual logged during a 2-week assessment period and examine differences in number of servings consumed between male and female participants. In this chapter, we will provide a step-by-step guide for using TVEM to estimate prevalence, means, and associations across age with a binary outcome and a count outcome. It is important to note that models with binary and count outcomes are interpreted in the same way as in generalized linear modeling (Agresti, 2015) but with the additional nuance of interpreting intercepts and associations as continuous functions of time or age.

This chapter will be divided into two sections. First, we will introduce generalized TVEM for a binary outcome and provide a detailed example of estimating the age-varying prevalence of a health outcome—having hypertension within the past year—as well as the age-varying associations of sex and racial/ethnic group and their interaction with past-year hypertension. Second, we will introduce generalized TVEM for a count outcome: the number of drinks reported during a typical drinking

S. T. Lanza, A. N. Linden-Carmichael, *Time-Varying Effect Modeling for the Behavioral, Social, and Health Sciences*,
https://doi.org/10.1007/978-3-030-70944-0_3

occasion in the past year. Here we will model the intercept as a continuous function of age and examine age-varying associations between sex and racial/ethnic group and their interaction with number of drinks.[1]

3.1 Part I. Generalized TVEM to Model Binary Outcomes

Similar to TVEM for continuous outcomes described in Chap. 2, generalized TVEM for binary outcomes, which we refer to here as logistic TVEM, can be used to examine regression coefficients (i.e., intercepts, slopes), and, therefore, odds and odds ratios, across continuous time. As noted in Chap. 2, intercept-only TVEM for continuous outcomes is used to estimate the mean level of a continuous variable, such as mean level of life satisfaction, across continuous age or time. This model is a direct extension of linear regression, where the intercept and slopes are estimated as a function of time. Binary outcomes are traditionally modeled using logistic regression to estimate the log-odds of an event occurring, with the outcome coded as 0 (the event did not occur) or 1 (the event did occur). The extension to TVEM is similarly direct, such that intercept-only time-varying effect models for binary outcomes are used to estimate the log-odds of an event—such as cardiovascular disease—occurring across continuous age or time. In traditional logistic regression, the intercept (and corresponding confidence interval) is exponentiated so that it can be interpreted as the odds of the event occurring; similarly, in logistic TVEM the intercept function (and corresponding confidence band) is exponentiated to facilitate interpretation. In this case, the exponentiated form of the intercept functions provide the time-varying or age-varying odds of the event occurring.

As an example, a researcher may be interested in understanding how odds of meeting physical activity guidelines (*PHYSACT*) change developmentally (i.e., across age). The researcher could use TVEM to model the **log-odds** (i.e., the natural log of the odds) of meeting the national guidelines, as follows:

$$ln\left(\frac{p\left(PHYSACT_i\right)}{1-p\left(PHYSACT_i\right)}\right)=\beta_0\left(t\right),$$

where ln refers to the natural logarithm, p refers to the probability, $PHYSACT_i$ represents whether individual i met the national guidelines, and $\beta_0(t)$ represents the estimated log-odds of meeting the national guidelines at a particular age. In traditional logistic regression, the intercept, β_0, would be a single-number estimate of the log-odds of meeting national guidelines for physical activity (among

[1]The special case of zero-inflated count outcomes is discussed briefly in Chap. 7. Zero-inflated models can be important when considering health conditions (e.g., number of diseases or conditions present) or behaviors (e.g., number of alcoholic drinks per week), as there can be an abundance of zeros in the count distribution. However, these models may be difficult to specify in such a way that the assumptions are plausible, and they can be computationally challenging to estimate.

individuals of all ages), but in logistic TVEM the intercept is estimated as a nonparametric function of time or age, allowing, in this example, the log-odds of meeting the national guidelines to vary flexibly across age.

By exponentiating the coefficient function, a more natural interpretation can be made—the **odds** of an individual meeting the guidelines for physical activity across age:

$$Odds\left(t\right) = e^{\beta_0(t)}.$$

For example, if three out of every four individuals meet the national guidelines (and, therefore, one out of every four does not), the odds of meeting guidelines are 3:1, or odds of 3.0. Understanding developmental changes in meeting national guidelines may be even more interpretable thus we can further transform the intercept function to consider the estimated **prevalence** of an event as follows:

$$Prevalence\left(t\right) = \frac{e^{\beta_0(t)}}{\left(1 + e^{\beta_0(t)}\right)}.$$

We obtain the estimated prevalence of the event in a population across age or time; often this transformation enables researchers to interpret the clinical significance of the finding. Continuing with the national guidelines for physical activity example, if three of every four individuals meet the national guidelines, that corresponds to 75%, or a prevalence of 0.75. In the context of TVEM, we would be able to interpret the proportion of individuals expected to meet national guidelines as a function of continuous age. We provide an empirical demonstration of this below, in which we estimate the prevalence of past-year hypertension across age.

Covariates can be incorporated in time-varying effect models for binary outcomes, as they can be when modeling continuous outcomes in TVEM. Findings would be interpreted in the same way as traditional logistic regression with an **odds ratio (OR)**, which expresses the change in odds of an event corresponding to a one-unit change on the covariate. As a brief review, logistic regression coefficients range from negative infinity to infinity, with a value of 0 corresponding to no association between the covariate and the event. Odds ratios, their exponentiated form, range from 0 to infinity, where an odds ratio of 1 corresponds to no expected change in the odds of the event corresponding to a one-unit increase on the covariate. An odds ratio greater than 1.0 is interpreted as the expected increase in odds of the event corresponding to a one-unit increase on the covariate; an odds ratio of less than 1.0 is interpreted as the expected decrease in odds of the event corresponding to a one-unit increase on the covariate. If an odds ratio is not statistically different from 1.0, this suggests that the covariate is not associated with the odds of the event occurring. For example, say we were interested in examining poverty (above the poverty line vs. at or below the poverty line) as a covariate in a model for meeting the national guidelines. Suppose we find that the odds of meeting the guidelines (i.e., a "success") is 4–1 for individuals above the poverty line and 2–1 for individuals below the poverty line. If we code poverty as 1 = above the poverty line and 0 = below the poverty line, our odds ratio is represented as

$$Odds\ ratio = \left[\frac{4/1}{2/1}\right] = 2.0.$$

This odds ratio of 2.0 implies that the odds of a success (i.e., meeting the national guidelines for physical activity) among individuals who are above the poverty line would be twice as high as the odds of success among individuals who are below the poverty line.

In TVEM, of course, we would interpret the association between the covariate and outcome as a function of continuous time or age; for example, we could examine the association between poverty and physical activity as a flexible function of age. When modeling longitudinal or intensive longitudinal data, covariates may be time-invariant or time-varying. As explained in Chap. 2, a time-invariant variable is one that typically does not change across time, such as an individual's racial/ethnic group or parent's education at baseline. Time-varying covariates may include variables such as current mood state or past-month physical activity. However, regardless of whether a covariate is time-invariant or time-varying, the *effect* of any covariate, or the association between any covariate and the outcome, may be specified to be constant over time/age (i.e., a time-invariant effect) or to vary across time/age (i.e., a time-varying effect). For example, although an individual's sex does not change across time, the association between physical activity and being male (coded as $MALE = 1$) relative to female (coded as $MALE = 0$) may vary across age:

$$ln\left(\frac{p(PHYSACT_i)}{1-p(PHYSACT_i)}\right) = \beta_0(t) + \beta_1(t)MALE_i,$$

where $PHYSACT_i$ represents whether individual i met national guidelines for physical activity, $\beta_0(t)$ is the intercept function representing the log-odds of female individuals meeting national guidelines across age, and $\beta_1(t)$ is the slope function, representing the change in log-odds of meeting national guidelines at each age for male individuals relative to female individuals.

When estimating the time-varying association between a binary covariate (e.g., sex) and a binary outcome (e.g., hypertension) using logistic TVEM, we recommend that the researcher examine both (1) the time-varying association of the covariate and the outcome to determine statistical significance (this slope is difficult to interpret because it is on the logit metric) and (2) the estimated prevalence of the outcome across time for each level of the covariate to enhance interpretability. For example, consider a model examining the association between being male (coded as 1 for male, 0 for female) and the odds of having high cholesterol (coded as 1 for meeting criteria for high cholesterol in the past year, 0 for not meeting criteria for high cholesterol in the past year) across ages 18–90. To test the association between being male and having high cholesterol, we would enter our variable *MALE* and specify that it has a time-varying effect.

The resultant coefficient function and confidence bands are then used to determine ages at which male adults have significantly different odds of having high cholesterol than female adults. The coefficient function for $\beta_1(t)$ can be used for this purpose, indicating significant sex differences for ages at which the confidence interval does not contain the value 0. Equivalently, the odds ratio function (i.e., the exponentiated coefficient function for the covariate *MALE*) can be used for significance testing by identifying ages at which the confidence interval does not contain the value 1. A significant positive effect at a particular age (i.e., OR > 1.0) would imply that male adults have greater odds than female adults at that age of having high cholesterol. For explanatory purposes, it is often helpful to plot the intercept function by first estimating the prevalence for only female adults (i.e., *MALE* = 0) and then reversing the coding of sex so that the intercept shows the estimated prevalence for male. In this way, the estimated prevalence of high cholesterol across age could be plotted for male and female adults, enabling an interpretation such as "at age 45, 20% of female and 30% of male adults had high cholesterol." The estimated prevalence for male and female adults can be plotted together, readily demonstrating how the estimated prevalence of high cholesterol fluctuates across age for each sex. If the data include sample weights, a **domain** statement can be used to restrict analysis to a subset of the data while retaining the full weighted sample. We demonstrate these approaches later in this chapter.

It is important to note that the hypothetical examples presented above are related to modeling binary outcomes across continuous age. As with TVEM for a continuous outcome, with logistic TVEM it also is possible to consider other metrics of time, including real-time and historical time. For example, in an ecological momentary assessment study following participants of a randomized, placebo-controlled trial of smoking cessation, Vasilenko et al. (2014) used logistic TVEM to estimate the odds of cigarette smoking during 14 consecutive days after a quit attempt. Here, participants completed multiple reports each day regarding their cravings and whether they smoked. Craving was entered as a time-varying covariate of smoking, with time coded as the length of time since actual quit date (continuously, from 0 to 14 days). Fig. 1 from the original paper, reproduced here as Fig. 3.1, shows the expected change in odds of smoking lapse corresponding to a one-unit increase in craving, as a function of time since quit date. Because the entire confidence band for the odds ratio is greater than 1.0 between days 1 and 13, we conclude that a higher level of craving was significantly associated with higher odds of a smoking lapse across most of the 14-day period. Further, the association between craving and relapse increased gradually from Day 1 to Day 12. The strongest significant association is observed around Day 12 when a one-unit increase in craving corresponds to twice the odds of relapse.

3.1.1 Example: Age-Varying Prevalence of Past-Year Hypertension and Associations With Sex and Racial/Ethnic Group

In this section, we walk through an empirical example modeling (1) past-year hypertension across age, (2) the age-varying associations of sex and racial/ethnic group with past-year hypertension, and (3) the interaction between sex and racial/ethnic group as related to past-year hypertension across age. Data are from the National Epidemiologic Survey on Alcohol and Related Conditions-III

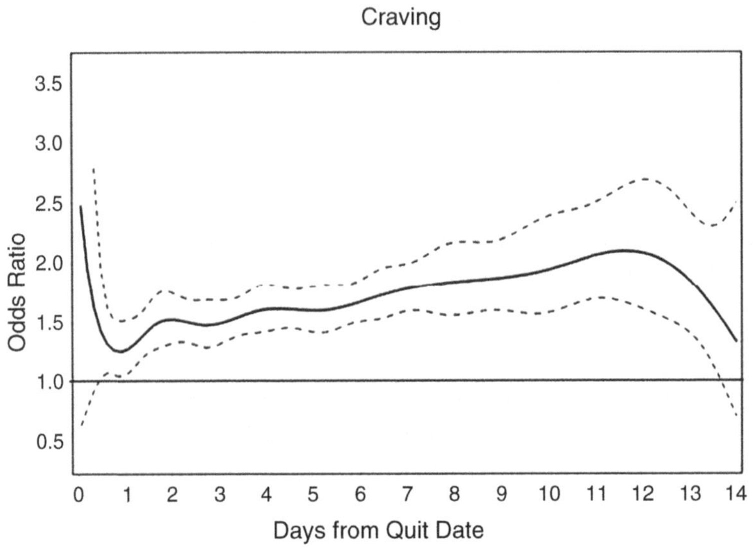

Fig. 3.1 Odds ratio corresponding to the change in odds of smoking lapse associated with a one-unit change in craving as a function of days since quit date, with corresponding 95% confidence band. Reproduced from Vasilenko, S. A., Piper, M. E., Lanza, S. T., Liu, X., Yang, J., and Li, R. (2014). Time-varying processes involved in smoking lapse in a randomized trial of smoking cessation therapies. Nicotine & Tobacco Research, 16(Suppl_2), S135-S143. By permission of the Society for Research on Nicotine and Tobacco

(NESARC-III; Grant et al., 2014), a nationally representative sample of more than 36,000 US adults aged 18 and older. Data from this cross-sectional study were collected in 2012 and 2013. Responses from Black, Hispanic/Latinx, and Asian adults were oversampled, so sample weights were used in all analyses and descriptive statistics. We restricted our analytic dataset to individuals who were between the ages of 18 and 80 ($n = 35{,}100$). Within this restricted sample, 51.6% of participants were female. Regarding racial/ethnic group, 65.5% were Non-Hispanic/Latinx White, 15.1% were Hispanic/Latinx, 12.0% were Non-Hispanic/Latinx Black, 5.8% were Non-Hispanic/Latinx Asian/Native Hawaiian/Other Pacific Islander, and 1.6% were Non-Hispanic/Latinx American Indian/Alaskan Native. Approximately one in four participants indicated that they had hypertension in the past year.

The primary variables for this analysis included sex, past-year hypertension, and racial/ethnic group. Sex was coded as 1 = male and 0 = female. Past-year hypertension was coded as 1 = yes and 0 = no (missing cases [$n = 163$] of past-year hypertension were excluded from analyses). We created dummy-coded indicators for racial/ethnic group, with Non-Hispanic/Latinx White as the reference group (the largest group; specified as the reference group to maximize statistical power in the estimates for pairwise group comparisons), including *BLACK* (1 = Non-Hispanic/Latinx Black, 0 = not Non-Hispanic/Latinx Black), *HISPANIC* (1 = Hispanic/Latinx, 0 = not Hispanic/Latinx), and *OTHER* (1 = Asian/Native Hawaiian/Other Pacific Islander and American Indian/Alaskan Native, 0 = not one of these groups).

For the purpose of this didactic example, we address the following research questions:

Research Question 1: What is the overall estimated prevalence of past-year hypertension across ages 18–80?

Research Question 2: How does the age-varying prevalence of past-year hypertension differ by sex and by racial/ethnic group? At what ages are there significant group differences?

Research Question 3: Do sex and racial/ethnic group interact to predict past-year hypertension? (In other words, do racial/ethnic group differences in hypertension across age differ by sex?)

3.1.2 *Research Question 1: What is the Overall Estimated Prevalence of Past-Year Hypertension Across Ages 18–80?*

An intercept-only model was used to estimate the log-odds of past-year hypertension across age. Results from this model can then be transformed to present age trends in the odds of past-year hypertension, then further transformed to present the estimated prevalence of hypertension (see equations above). The intercept-only model specified here is

$$ln\left(\frac{p(HIGHBP_i)}{1+p(HIGHBP_i}\right)=\beta_0(t),$$

where hypertension ($HIGHBP_i$) is a dummy-coded variable indicating whether individual i reported hypertension (coded as 1 = yes, 0 = no) and $\beta_0(t)$ is the coefficient function for the log-odds of hypertension across continuous age. To estimate this model, we specified the following %WeightedTVEM macro statement in SAS:

```
%WeightedTVEM(
data = nesarc_chapter3a,
dist = binary,
cluster = caseid,
time = nage,
dv = highbp,
tvary_effect = int,
knots = 1,
weight = audweight);
```

Because the outcome is dichotomous, we specify the distribution to be "binary" for our **dist** statement. The **data** statement indicates the name of our working dataset. The **cluster** statement refers to our participant ID variable; because this is a cross-sectional dataset, each row in our vertical dataset represents each unique participant's responses. **Time** refers to how we specify time on the *x*-axis; in this case, time is considered participants' age, stored in a variable denoted *NAGE*. **DV** is the outcome of interest; here, our outcome is whether individuals met criteria for past-year hypertension, labeled *HIGHBP*. Because this simple model evaluates only the estimated log-odds of the dependent variable (*HIGHBP*) across age and does not estimate any time-varying associations with blood pressure, our **tvary_effect** will include only the intercept. We have already created a variable in our dataset (called *INT*) which is equal to 1 for all rows of data to facilitate estimation of the intercept function.

Our **knots** statement refers to the number of splitting points we are specifying for the intercept coefficient function, with a higher number of knots corresponding to a more complex function. As noted in Chap. 2, because our analysis uses weighted data, we must use B-spline modeling. B-spline modeling requires the user to specify the number of knots; thus, the user must conduct model selection manually by comparing the relative fit of models with different numbers of knots. Because this simple model only estimates the intercept as a function of time, we only need to specify the number of knots for a single coefficient function. We ran our intercept-only model five times, each with a different specified number of knots for the intercept function. We suggest starting with the most complex model to be considered and reduce complexity systematically. In this example, we began with specifying 5 knots, corresponding to a more complex function, then decreased the number of knots one at a time until we reached 1 knot, corresponding to a less complex function. We then compared the Akaike information criterion (AIC) and the Bayesian information criterion (BIC) for each model. The AIC and BIC values for each model with 1 through 5 knots are specified in Table 3.1.

The AIC and BIC values are both lowest in the one-knot model, representing an optimal balance between model fit and parsimony for the model with only one knot specified (minimum values are bolded in Table 3.1 for emphasis). Thus, we will specify **1** for the final **knots** statement for this model, corresponding to a function that is relatively less complex. Lastly, our model specifies the name of our **weight** variable, *AUDWEIGHT*, which was already created for this dataset and is used to ensure that the findings are more representative of the population. We note that the **method** statement is not available for weighted TVEM because B-spline is the only spline estimation option.

Table 3.1 Model fit information for selecting the optimal number of knots for the intercept function

Model #	# Knots for *INT*	AIC	BIC
1	5	32305.93	32382.08
2	4	32304.21	32371.90
3	3	32306.15	32365.38
4	2	32304.44	32355.21
5	**1**	**32302.47**	**32344.78**

For logistic TVEM, the default output includes a plot of the coefficient function for the log-odds and a plot showing the exponentiated values of $\beta_0(t)$, reflecting the estimated odds across age to facilitate interpretation. This exponentiated intercept function represents the estimated odds of hypertension across age, along with corresponding 95% confidence bands. To obtain a more interpretable prevalence, we further transformed the coefficient function using the formula for the prevalence function, described in detail below. A plot of the transformed coefficient function for $\beta_0(t)$, presented in Fig. 3.2, shows how the estimated prevalence of hypertension changes over continuous age from 18 to 80 years, with corresponding 95% confidence bands.

Several SAS datasets are automatically stored in the SAS Work directory. As noted in Chap. 2, values from the estimated coefficient functions are stored in the dataset **tvem_plot_data**. When specifying a binary outcome in logistic TVEM, odds ratios are provided in the **tvem_plot_data_or** dataset. This dataset is similar to **tvem_plot_data,** but it includes exponentiated coefficients. These datasets contain the information that was used to produce the default figures (for the time-varying log-odds and odds) shown in the SAS output. Similar to procedures in Chap. 2, estimated coefficients were exported into Excel to facilitate figure creation. The companion website for this book (https://prevention.psu.edu/books/tvem/) provides didactic information on creating figures of coefficient functions in Excel using the default SAS output.

Returning to our example, we first run the %WeightedTVEM macro syntax for the intercept-only model, which generates the **tvem_plot_data_or** dataset. To convert the odds of past-year hypertension to more interpretable prevalence of

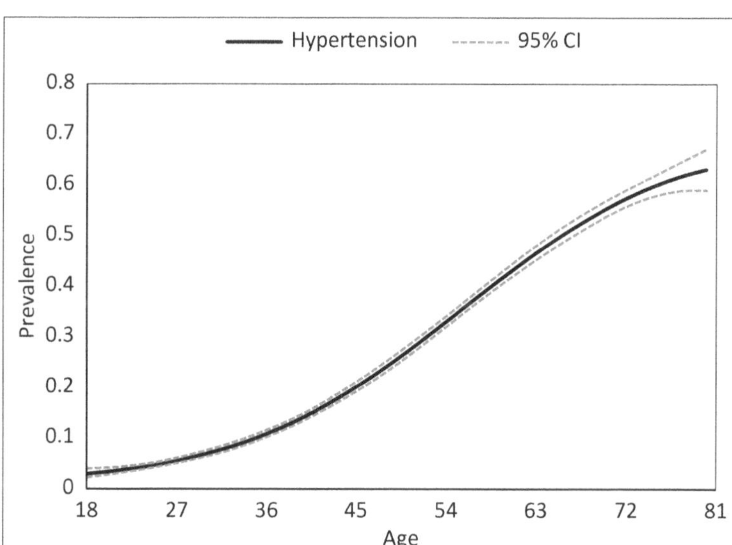

Fig. 3.2 Estimated prevalence of past-year hypertension across age

past-year hypertension, we create a new dataset name (we call it **highbp** here) derived from the **tvem_plot_data_or** dataset. Within this new dataset, we use the exponentiated intercept (*exp_INT*), which is the estimated odds of hypertension, and its associated confidence intervals (*exp_INT_l* for lower-bound of confidence interval and *exp_INT_u* for the upper-bound of confidence interval) to calculate the estimated prevalence of past-year hypertension. To do this, we simply divide the exponentiated intercept (*exp_INT*) by 1 plus the exponentiated intercept (1 + *exp_INT*). We will do the same for the lower and upper bounds of the exponentiated intercept. The following SAS syntax creates a new dataset called **highbp** that contains the newly calculated prevalence estimate (in variable *HPROP*) and corresponding confidence interval values (in variables *HPROP_L* and *HPROP_U* for lower and upper bounds, respectively) across the age range:

```
data highbp;
set tvem_plot_data_or;
hprop = exp_int/(1+exp_int);
hprop_l = exp_int_l/(1+exp_int_l);
hprop_u = exp_int_u/(1+exp_int_u);
run;
```

Next, we export the SAS working dataset called **highbp** to Excel as follows:

```
PROC EXPORT DATA=highbp DBMS=xlsx
OUTFILE="C:\FolderName\highbp.xlsx";
run;
```

When opened in Excel, the first several rows of data will be displayed, as shown in Table 3.2.

Table 3.2 First several rows of data contained in the tvem_plot_data_or dataset

nage	exp_int_L	exp_int	exp_int_U	exp_int_SE	hprop	hprop_l	hprop_u
18	0.02204	0.03015	0.04125	1.17342	0.02927	0.02156	0.03961
18.6263	0.02375	0.03146	0.04167	1.15419	0.03050	0.02320	0.04000
19.2525	0.02555	0.03285	0.04224	1.13689	0.03181	0.02491	0.04053
19.8788	0.02742	0.03432	0.04297	1.12142	0.03319	0.02669	0.04120
20.5051	0.02936	0.03588	0.04385	1.10772	0.03464	0.02853	0.04201
21.1313	0.03138	0.03753	0.04490	1.09574	0.03618	0.03042	0.04297
21.7576	0.03345	0.03928	0.04613	1.08542	0.03780	0.03237	0.04409
22.3838	0.03558	0.04113	0.04754	1.07671	0.03950	0.03436	0.04538
23.0101	0.03777	0.04309	0.04916	1.06955	0.04131	0.03639	0.04685
23.6364	0.04000	0.04516	0.05098	1.06386	0.04321	0.03846	0.04851
24.2626	0.04227	0.04735	0.05303	1.05952	0.04521	0.04056	0.05036
24.8889	0.04460	0.04966	0.05530	1.05636	0.04731	0.04270	0.05240
25.5152	0.04699	0.05212	0.05780	1.05420	0.04953	0.04488	0.05464
26.1414	0.04946	0.05471	0.06051	1.05280	0.05187	0.04713	0.05706

NAGE is the time axis representing participants' age. Values range from 18 to 80, with 100 equally spaced intervals across that age range. *HPROP* is the exponentiated proportion of individuals at each respective age who have reported past-year hypertension (i.e., the estimated age-varying prevalence). *HPROP_L* and *HPROP_U* represent the associated lower and upper bound of the confidence intervals for *HPROP*, respectively. To create a figure in Excel reflecting TVEM results, graph *HPROP*, *HPROP_L*, and *HPROP_U* along the *x*-axis of *NAGE*. More details and a demonstration of graphing TVEM results in Excel are presented on the companion website for this book (https://prevention.psu.edu/books/tvem/). Figure 3.2 shows the prevalence of past-year hypertension across age. The solid black line represents the estimated coefficient function and the dashed lines on either side of the estimate represent the associated 95% confidence bands. As can be seen here, the prevalence increases fairly steadily across age, ranging from 0.029 (~3%) at age 18 to its highest level at age 80, with 0.631 (~63%) of 80-year-olds sampled indicating past-year hypertension.

3.1.3 Research Question 2: How Does the Age-Varying Prevalence of Past-Year Hypertension Differ by Sex and by Racial/Ethnic Group? At What Ages are There Significant Group Differences?

Next, covariates are added to estimate the age-varying associations of sex and racial/ethnic group with past-year hypertension. We first estimate the age-varying association of sex—indicated here with the variable *MALE* (1 = male, 0 = female)—with hypertension across ages 18–80. The syntax is generally the same as that presented in Research Question 1, with two modifications:

```
%WeightedTVEM(
data = nesarc_chapter3a,
dist = binary,
cluster = caseid,
time = nage,
dv = highbp,
tvary_effect = int male,
knots = 1 1,
weight=audweight);
```

The first difference from the model presented above is that we have added *MALE* as a covariate on the **tvary_effect** line of syntax in addition to the intercept (*INT*, which is the variable containing the value 1 for all records). This will produce two age-varying coefficient functions, one for the intercept and one for the coefficient for male. The second difference is that we added a second specification for the number of **knots**. Because we are now estimating two coefficient functions, we need to specify the number of knots for each. The decision to specify 1 knot for each function is described next.

3.1.3.1 Model Selection

To determine the appropriate number of knots, we first tested the appropriate number of knots for *MALE* and then the appropriate number of knots for *INT*. Following an approach to model selection that has worked well in practice, we start with 5 knots for both *MALE* and *INT*, then decrease the number of knots for male while keeping the number of knots for *INT* constant at 5. As shown in Table 3.3 (selected number of knots bolded for emphasis), after decreasing the number of knots for *MALE* the optimal knot selection for *MALE* is 1. Thus, we will keep the number of knots at 1 for *MALE* and then test the number of knots most appropriate for *INT*. We begin at 5 knots for *INT* (Model 5), decreasing the number of knots in each subsequent model. As indicated by minimum AIC and BIC values, the optimal number of knots for *MALE* and *INT* is 1 knot each thus we select Model 9 as our final model. In this example, the model selection procedure resulted in selecting a number of knots for each coefficient function that corresponds to curves with relatively less complexity. Thus, neither the intercept function nor the effect of being male showed extreme fluctuations in the estimated effect across continuous age. However, coefficient functions with 1 knot still can convey considerably more nuance across age than, say, linear functions.

After running the TVEM macro syntax, we will examine the odds ratio plot showing the difference in odds of hypertension for male versus female adults (this information also stored in **tvem_plot_data_or**), as shown in Fig. 3.3a. The solid black line represents the odds ratio associated with being male across age, and the dashed lines represent the associated 95% confidence band across age. The estimate indicates the difference in odds of past-year hypertension for male adults relative to female adults at each age. The confidence intervals here indicate whether the

Table 3.3 Model fit information for selecting the optimal number of knots for the intercept and slope coefficient functions

Model #	# Knots for *INT*	# Knots for *MALE*	AIC	BIC
1	5	5	32274.35	32426.65
2	5	4	32274.36	32418.20
3	5	3	32274.99	32410.37
4	5	2	32273.37	32400.29
5	5	1	32271.50	32389.96
6	4	1	32269.74	32379.74
7	3	1	32271.83	32373.36
8	2	1	32270.31	32363.39
9	**1**	**1**	**32268.20**	**32352.81**

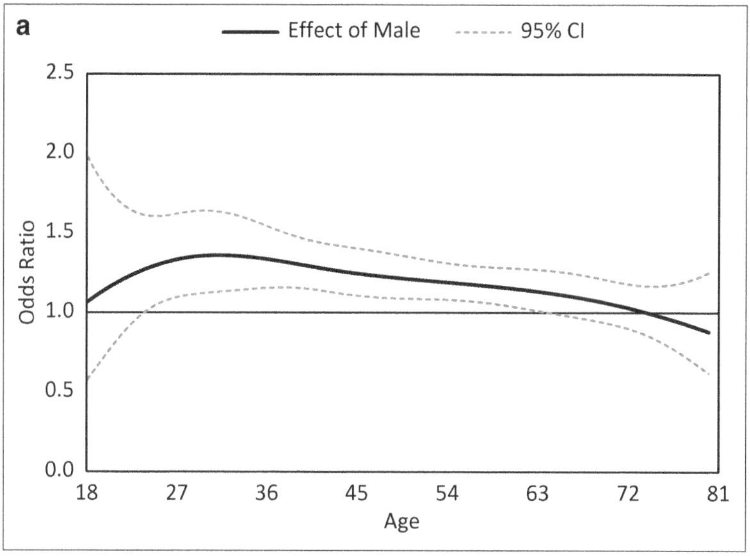

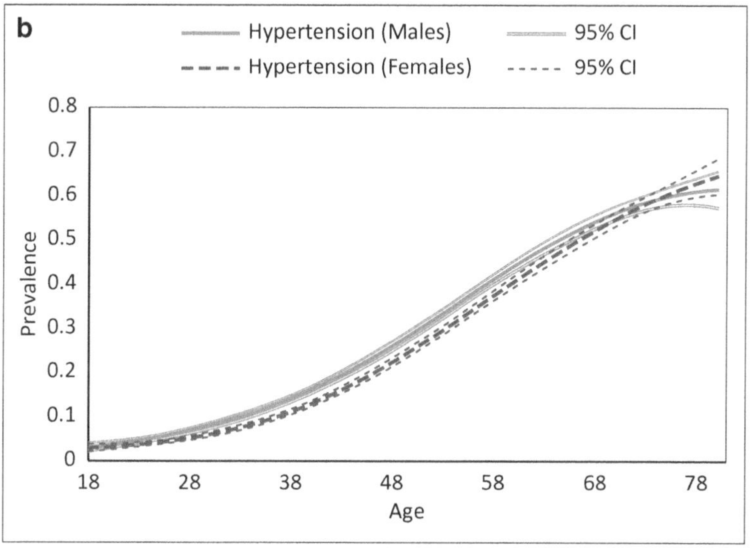

Fig. 3.3 (**a**) Odds ratio corresponding to the change in odds of hypertension associated with being male across age. (**b**) Estimated prevalence of past-year hypertension and corresponding 95% confidence interval across age, separately by male (solid green line) and female (dashed purple line)

association between sex and the odds of past-year hypertension is significant at each age. Because an odds ratio of 1.0 indicates no association between the covariate and the outcome, we can examine ages at which the confidence interval does not overlap with 1.0 to determine statistical significance. As shown in Fig. 3.3a, from approximately ages 24–62 the confidence intervals do not include 1.0 and the estimate is above 1.0. This indicates that between the ages of 24 and 62, male adults are at significantly higher odds of past-year hypertension relative to female adults, with the odds ratio peaking at roughly age 31 (OR = 1.36, CI = 1.13–1.64). Although we see the estimated odds ratio fall below 1.0 in later ages, specifically ages 75–80, the confidence intervals contain the value 1.0 and thus we fail to reject the null hypothesis of no association between sex and hypertension.

3.1.3.2 Interpreting Odds Ratio Functions: Calculating Group-Specific Prevalences

It can further aid interpretation to plot the prevalence of past-year hypertension across age separately by sex. To produce these plots, we will need to slightly modify our syntax. Because we are using the %WeightedTVEM macro, we have the option to add **domain** and **which** statements that will generate plots for each level of the covariate. The **domain** statement specifies the covariate to be used (in this case, *MALE*), and the **which** statement specifies the level of the domain variable to be plotted. This is an extremely useful approach for understanding associations between a categorical covariate and an outcome over time. We note that the domain variable can have 2 or more categories. Here we show syntax that generates a plot of the estimated odds of hypertension among male adults only (*MALE* = 1):

```
%WeightedTVEM(
data = nesarc_chapter3a,
dist =binary,
cluster = caseid,
time = nage,
dv = highbp,
tvary_effect = int,
knots = 1,
weight=audweight,
domain = male,
which = 1);
```

First, we will produce the same %WeightedTVEM macro syntax but remove male from the list of time-varying effects to be estimated (and the corresponding knot value for the effect of male). We then add a **domain** statement, which is the name of the domain variable for restricting analysis to a subset of the data. We indicate that the domain variable of interest is *MALE*. We then add another line of syntax specifying the **which** statement; here, we specify the level of the domain variable (*MALE*) we wish to examine. First, we run the macro specifying "**which** = 1" to obtain the results for male adults; we then specify "**which** = 0" and rerun the macro to obtain the results for female adults. This approach allows the sample weights to be applied appropriately while examining results only for a subgroup of individuals.

Similar to calculating the prevalence of past-year hypertension overall, we can also calculate prevalence among male adults. To do this, we use the TVEM plot data produced from specifying the level of the **which** argument: **tvem_1_plot_data_or**. Note that the filename now includes "1" indicating the level on the domain variable being examined. We choose to rename this dataset by creating a dataset called **highbp_male**. Then, we calculate the proportion of male adults (*MPROP*) with past-year hypertension (i.e., the prevalence among male adults) and corresponding confidence interval for male adults, across age. Finally, we export our male dataset into Excel for plotting purposes.

```
data highbp_male;
set tvem_1_plot_data_or;
mprop=exp_int/(1+exp_int);
mprop_l=exp_int_l/(1+exp_int_l);
mprop_u=exp_int_u/(1+exp_int_u);
run;

PROC EXPORT DATA=highbp_male DBMS=xlsx
OUTFILE="C:\FolderName\highbp_male.xlsx";
run;
```

Next, we modify our model specification and rerun the %WeightedTVEM macro, this time specifying the analyses to reflect only the female domain. To do this, we simply change the level of the variable *MALE* in the **which** statement; we now request model results for female adults only (indicated in the data by *MALE* = 0).

```
%WeightedTVEM(
data = nesarc_chapter3a,
dist =binary,
cluster = caseid,
time = nage,
dv = highbp,
tvary_effect = int,
knots = 1,
weight=audweight,
domain = male,
which = 0);
```

As we did for male adults, we transform the model results into prevalences by first creating a new dataset with the automatically generated dataset for female adults: **tvem_0_plot_data_or**. Again, this dataset is automatically denoted with "0" in the dataset name because of the level specified for the domain variable *MALE*. As shown below, we will create a new dataset (**highbp_female**) and name our proportion variable (i.e., the prevalence among female adults) for female adults *FPROP*.

```
data highbp_female
set tvem_0_plot_data_or;
fprop=exp_int/(1+exp_int);
fprop_l=exp_int_l/(1+exp_int_l);
fprop_u=exp_int_u/(1+exp_int_u);
run;

PROC EXPORT DATA=highbp_female DBMS=xlsx
OUTFILE="C:\FolderName\highbp_female.xlsx"
run;
```

After running the syntax and exporting the data file, we merge the male and female files, matching the time variable (*NAGE* in this case). (Equivalently, we could have merged the **highbp_male** and **highbp_female** datasets in SAS and then exported a single dataset to Excel.) We then create a plot with age on the *x*-axis, showing the male proportion variable and associated confidence intervals (*MPROP*, *MPROP_L*, and *MPROP_U*) and the female proportion variable and associated confidence intervals (*FPROP*, *FPROP_L*, and *FPROP_U*). This will generate a plot as shown in Fig. 3.3b. Here, the solid green line and associated confidence intervals represent the estimated prevalence of past-year hypertension among male adults across ages 18–80. The dashed purple line represents the estimated prevalence of past-year hypertension among female adults across age. Male and female adults show a very similar age trend in the prevalence, gradually increasing across age; male adults have a slightly higher prevalence of hypertension across most ages in middle adulthood, particularly throughout the late 20s through the 50s. As noted above, Fig. 3.3a should be relied upon to test the hypothesis for age-varying sex differences in the odds of hypertension (Fig. 3.3a). Recall our conclusion from Fig. 3.3a, that male adults had significantly higher odds of hypertension between ages 24 and 62. It is tempting to simply rely on Fig. 3.3b to visualize ages at which odds of hypertension differ significantly by sex, for example, by identifying ages at which the confidence intervals for the two groups do not overlap. We caution against making statistical inferences based on ages at which confidence intervals for prevalence between groups do not overlap however as this may be an overly conservative estimate. Our recommendation is to test for statistical significance between groups by examining the time-varying effect of a covariate across age and determining ages at which the confidence interval for the effect (i.e., the odds ratio, as shown in Fig. 3.3a) does not include 1.0. The **tvem_plot_data_or** dataset can be examined to identify precise ages at which the confidence intervals of the odds ratio do not contain 1, if such precision is desired. For readership purposes, it is often easier for the reader to view differences between groups as shown in Fig. 3.3b. Thus, it could be stated in the Results section of a manuscript that age regions of significance were determined by examining the time-varying effect of a covariate (*MALE*) on an outcome (*HYPERTENSION*), but weighted prevalences are provided separately by group to facilitate interpretation.

For the purpose of this didactic example, we also tested the prevalence of past-year hypertension by racial/ethnic group. Because there are multiple groups represented, we tested the time-varying effect of racial/ethnic group by including dummy

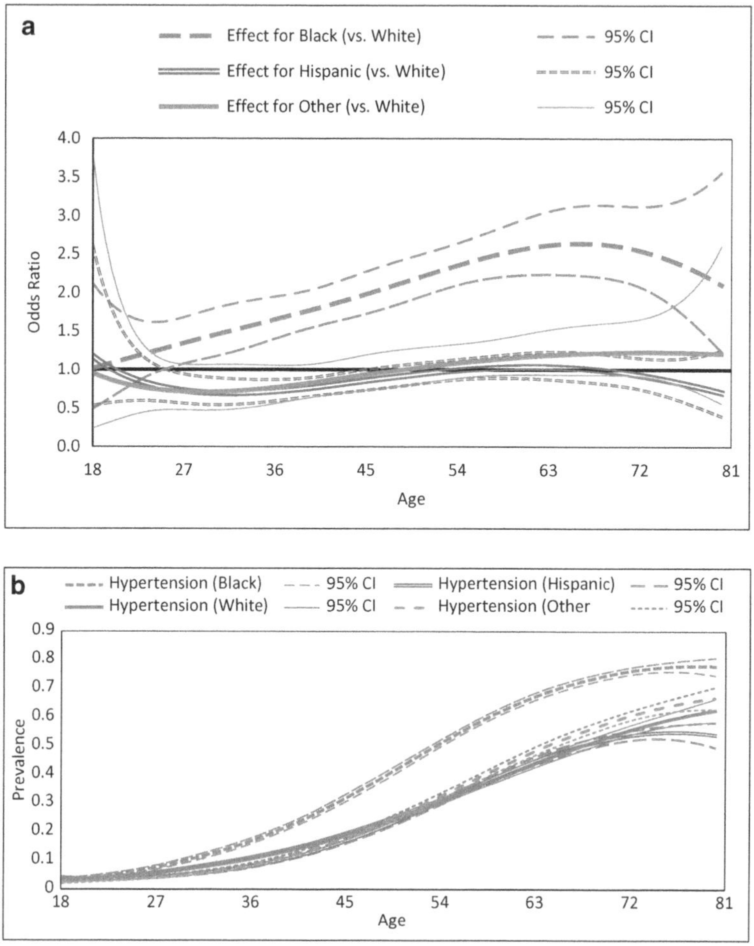

Fig. 3.4 (**a**) Odds ratio corresponding to the change in odds of hypertension associated with being Black, Hispanic/Latinx, or Other racial/ethnic group relative to White adults across ages 18–80. (**b**) Estimated prevalence of past-year hypertension across age separately for Black, Hispanic/Latinx, White, and Other racial/ethnic groups of adults

codes for Non-Hispanic/Latinx Black, Hispanic/Latinx, and Other adults (with Non-Hispanic/Latinx White adults as our reference). Consistent with our procedures for examining sex, we conducted weighted TVEM by specifying each dummy-coded indicator as having a time-varying effect on past-year hypertension. Significant differences were detected for Non-Hispanic/Latinx Black and Hispanic/Latinx adults relative to Non-Hispanic/Latinx White adults on odds of past-year hypertension (odds ratios shown in Fig. 3.4a), so we proceeded to use the **domain** and **which** statements to separately plot the estimated prevalence of past-year hypertension across age, separately for Non-Hispanic/Latinx White, Non-Hispanic/Latinx Black, Hispanic/Latinx, and "Other" adults (prevalences shown in Fig. 3.4b).

As shown in Fig. 3.4b, Non-Hispanic/Latinx White (solid green line), Hispanic/Latinx (double purple line), and "Other" individuals (long-dashed blue line) had similar prevalences of past-year hypertension, with a small but significantly higher prevalence among Non-Hispanic/Latinx White adults compared to Hispanic/Latinx adults during the 30s and early 40s. The prevalence of hypertension was substantially higher among Non-Hispanic/Latinx Black adults (short-dashed orange line) than the other racial/ethnic groups from the late 20s through age 80. Prevalence peaked among all groups at age 80 with 77.7% of Non-Hispanic/Latinx Black adults, 62.4% of Non-Hispanic/Latinx White adults, 53.9% of Hispanic/Latinx adults, and 66.7% of adults belonging to the "Other" group reporting past-year hypertension.

3.1.4 *Research Question 3: Do Sex and Racial/Ethnic Group Interact to Predict Past-Year Hypertension? (In Other Words, Do Racial/Ethnic Group Differences in Hypertension Across Age Differ by Sex?)*

To address the last research question, we tested the interaction effect of sex and racial/ethnic group on the odds of past-year hypertension across age. As in a standard regression model, the model should include an intercept (*INT*), main effects including sex (*male*) and racial/ethnic group dummy codes (*BLACK*, *HISPANIC*, *OTHER*), and three interaction terms we created for sex by each racial/ethnic group (*SEX_BLACK*, *SEX_HISP*, *SEX_OTHER*). Each of these variable names will be listed under the **tvary_effect** argument to allow any moderation effect to vary flexibly across age.

```
%WeightedTVEM(
data = nesarc_chapter3a,
dist =binary,
cluster = caseid,
time = nage,
dv = highbp,
tvary_effect = int male Black Hispanic Other
Sex_Black Sex_Hisp Sex_Other,
knots = 1 1 1 1 1 1 1 1,
weight=audweight);
```

Consistent with the model selection procedure demonstrated above, one value for the number of knots is specified for each time-varying effect. The appropriate number of knots were tested for each variable, beginning with 5 knots each and first selecting the optimal number of knots for each interaction term, then each main effect, then finally the intercept. Using this approach, we selected 1 knot per coefficient function. The coefficient functions that allow us to test for moderation are the plots for the effects of *SEX_BLACK*, *SEX_HISP*, and *SEX_OTHER*, found in the **tvem_plot_data** working dataset. When modeling interactions, either the β coefficient curve (where a value of 0 indicates no association) or the odds ratio curve (where a value of 1 indicates no association) may be used for testing the significance of an interaction term; neither is easily interpreted in this context. Because the β coefficients can be used to calculate simple slopes that will aid in interpretation, we recommend using the β coefficient curve when testing significance for interaction terms. Figure 3.5 shows the statistical significance of interaction terms across continuous age. These plots represent the time-varying effects of the interaction of sex and each racial/ethnic group in predicting the log-odds of past-year hypertension. As indicated by confidence intervals that do not include 0, the interaction for male by Non-Hispanic/Latinx Black on odds of hypertension is statistically significant from ages 21 to 46 and from ages 54 to 73 (Fig. 3.5a).[2] The interaction for male by Hispanic on hypertension is significant from ages 34 to 40 and from ages 53 to 71 (Fig. 3.5b). The sex by Other racial/ethnic group interaction term was not statistically significant at any age, indicating that the age-varying effect of sex did not differ between adults in the Non-Hispanic/Latinx White and Other racial/ethnic groups (Fig. 3.5c).

Similar to a standard regression where interaction terms are best understood by examining simple slopes, it is helpful in TVEM to interpret the interaction term by plotting the effect of one variable within each group. Thus, we examined the simple slope, or the effect of sex on past-year hypertension, separately for Non-Hispanic/Latinx White, Non-Hispanic/Latinx Black, and Hispanic/Latinx adults. To do this, we specified our **tvary_effect** for our intercept (*INT*) and the effect of sex (*MALE*), with a number of knots specified for each. We then specified a **domain** statement for our race variable (*NETHRACE*), which is coded as 1 = Non-Hispanic/Latinx White, 2 = Non-Hispanic/Latinx Black, and 3 = Hispanic/Latinx.[3] To first examine the effect of sex among Non-Hispanic/Latinx White adults, we ran the following syntax:

```
%WeightedTVEM(
data = nesarc_chapter3a,
dist = binary,
cluster = caseid,
time = nage,
dv = highbp,
tvary_effect = int male,
knots = 1 1,
weight = audweight,
domain = nethrace,
which = 1);
```

[2] Especially in cases where the confidence intervals hover close to 0, it is helpful to check the generated dataset for the precise 95% confidence interval at each age.

[3] The effect of sex among Other racial/ethnic groups was not further explored because the main interaction term of sex by Other racial/ethnic group was nonsignificant.

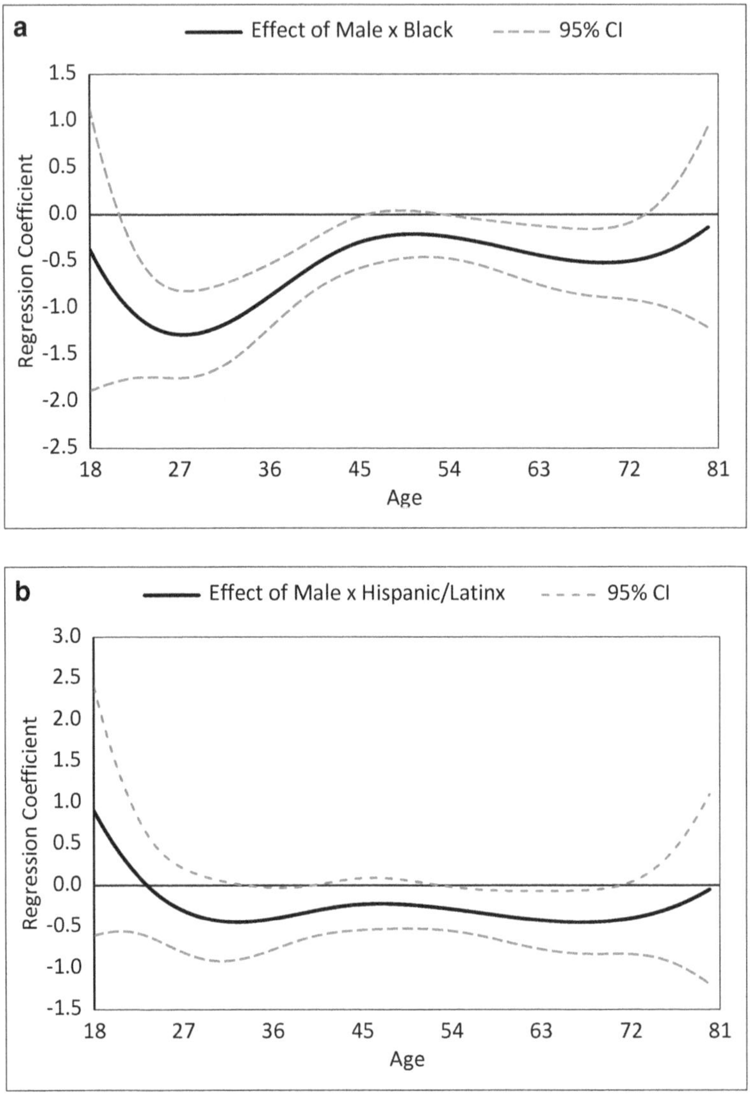

Fig. 3.5 Coefficient functions corresponding to the interaction between the indicator of being male and indicators of being (**a**) Black, (**b**) Hispanic/Latinx, and (**c**) Other racial/ethnic group on past-year hypertension across age

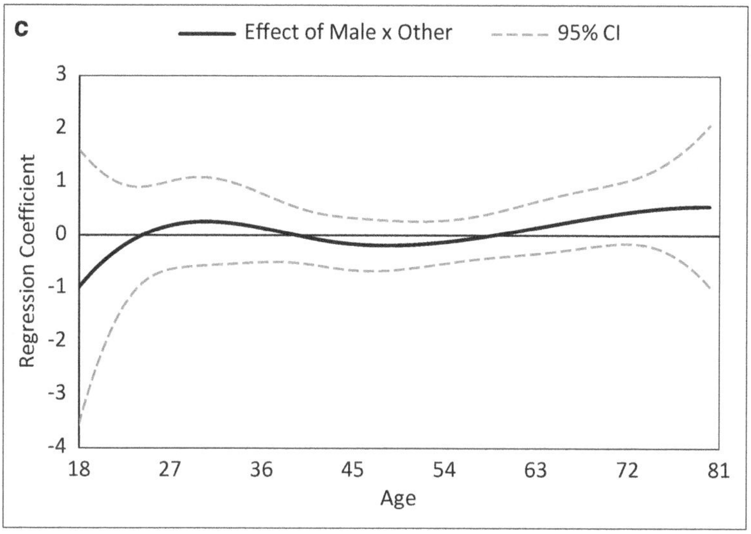

Fig. 3.5 (continued)

As Non-Hispanic/Latinx White adults were coded as *NETHRACE* = 1, the **which** statement was set to 1 and the dataset **tvem_1_plot_data_or** was saved as a SAS dataset we renamed as **sexonbp_white**. This procedure was repeated two times, once specifying the effect of sex among Non-Hispanic/Latinx Black adults (**which** = 2) and once specifying the effect of sex among Hispanic/Latinx adults (**which** = 3). The coefficients for *MALE* for each racial/ethnic group across age were combined (i.e., merged) by matching on the time variable (*NAGE*, in this case) so that the coefficient functions and their corresponding confidence bands could be plotted simultaneously. The syntax used to generate each model and the Excel data used to create figures for the curves within each group are available on the companion website for this book (https://prevention.psu.edu/books/tvem/).

Figure 3.6 shows the odds ratios across ages 18–80 corresponding to the change in odds of past-year hypertension for male adults relative to female adults among Non-Hispanic/Latinx Black adults (long-dashed orange line), Hispanic/Latinx adults (double purple line), and Non-Hispanic/Latinx White (solid green line) adults. There are two key pieces of information to process: the overall significance of the effect of sex on past-year hypertension within each racial/ethnic group (i.e., ages at which the respective confidence intervals for the effect of being male do not include 1.0) and differences between groups (i.e., ages at which the confidence intervals for each group do not overlap). We noted above that one should draw inference based on the overlap (or lack of overlap) of confidence intervals across groups cautiously, as it can be an overly conservative test of group differences. This is not a precise test of statistical significance of the group difference, and the approach may lead one to miss other ages at which a group difference is in fact statistically significant.

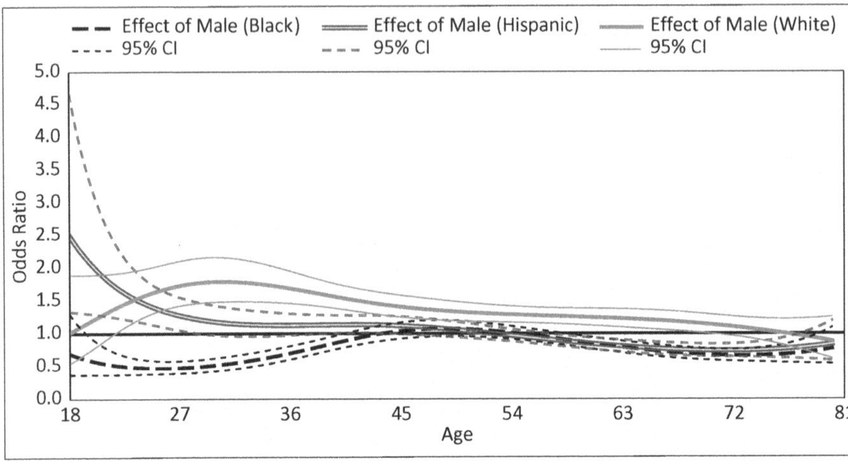

Fig. 3.6 Age-varying odds ratios showing the effect of being male on past-year hypertension among Black, Hispanic/Latinx, and White adults

When examining the effect of sex on hypertension for each racial/ethnic group, we see that among Non-Hispanic/Latinx White adults, the effect of sex on hypertension is statistically significant from ages 22 to 70, indicating that male adults are at increased risk for past-year hypertension relative to female adults at these ages. For Non-Hispanic/Latinx Black adults, the effect of sex is significant from ages 20 to 40 and from ages 59 to 79, but the odds are less than 1.0, indicating that male Non-Hispanic/Latinx Black adults are at lower risk for past-year hypertension at these ages than female Non-Hispanic/Latinx Black adults. Lastly, the effect of sex for Hispanic adults is significant and greater than 1.0 from ages 18 to 29 and ages 39–44 and significant and less than 1.0 from ages 57 to 77. Thus, male (vs. female) Hispanic/Latinx individuals are at higher risk for past-year hypertension in young and middle adulthood, but female (vs. male) Hispanic/Latinx adults are at higher risk in their late 50s through late 70s. Differences between groups can also be examined, albeit approximately, by comparing coefficient functions and corresponding confidence intervals between groups. For example, the effect of sex for Non-Hispanic/Latinx Black adults relative to Hispanic/Latinx adults is smaller from approximately ages 18 to 40 and, relative to Non-Hispanic/Latinx White adults, the effect of sex is lower from approximately ages 20 to 46 and again from ages 56 to 74. This approach presents an optimal way of interpreting time-varying moderation effects in TVEM, but an optimal way to test whether, say, the association of sex with hypertension differs between Non-Hispanic/Latinx Black and Hispanic/Latinx adults, would involve additional dummy coding and specifying the appropriate reference group (e.g., with Non-Hispanic/Latinx adults as the reference group).

3.1.5 Sample Results Section

Sample Results Section: Past-Year Hypertension

Research Question 1. The estimated prevalence of past-year hypertension is presented in Fig. 3.1. Overall prevalence increased fairly smoothly across ages 18–80. The estimated prevalence was lowest at age 18, with 3.0% of 18-year-olds reporting past-year hypertension, and were highest at age 80, with 63.1% in this age group reporting hypertension.

Research Question 2. The estimated prevalences of past-year hypertension by sex are shown in Fig. 3.3b. Male (solid green line) and female (dashed purple line) adults followed a similar pattern with the prevalence increasing fairly linearly across age. To determine whether sex differences in the prevalence were statistically significant, sex was included as a predictor of past-year hypertension and specified to have an age-varying effect. Findings revealed that male adults were at significantly greater odds of meeting criteria for past-year hypertension from ages 24 to 62 (largest OR observed at age 31 = 1.36, CI = 1.13–1.64). This sex difference was statistically significant but relatively small, with the largest difference observed at age 39 showing that 15.3% of male and 12.2% of female adults reported past-year hypertension.

Differences in racial/ethnic group also were tested by entering three dummy-coded indicators of racial/ethnic group (Non-Hispanic/Latinx Black, Hispanic/Latinx, Other) with Non-Hispanic/Latinx White as the reference group. Group differences in past-year hypertension were specified as age-varying. Differences in the prevalence of past-year hypertension for Non-Hispanic/Latinx White, Non-Hispanic/Latinx Black, Hispanic/Latinx, and Other adults are shown in Fig. 3.4b. Non-Hispanic/Latinx White (solid green line), Hispanic/Latinx (double purple line), and Other adults (long-dashed blue line) had similar rates of past-year hypertension, but the prevalence was much higher among Non-Hispanic/Latinx Black adults (short-dashed orange line) from the late 20s through age 80. The prevalence peaked among all groups at age 80, with approximately 77.7% of Non-Hispanic/Latinx Black, 62.4% of Non-Hispanic/Latinx White, 53.9% of Hispanic/Latinx, and 66.7% of Other adults reporting past-year hypertension.

Research Question 3. Finally, we modeled the interaction of sex and racial/ethnic group and their main effects on the odds of past-year hypertension across age. Assessment of the interaction terms revealed a positive, significant interaction for Non-Hispanic/Latinx Black adults from ages 21 to 46 and ages 54 to 73. The interaction term was significant for Hispanic/Latinx adults from ages 34 to 40 and from ages 53 to 71. The interaction term was nonsignificant for Other adults across all ages.

To further explore the interaction, we plotted the effect of being male within each racial/ethnic group. Figure 3.6 shows the effect of sex among Non-Hispanic/Latinx Black (long-dashed orange line), Hispanic/Latinx (double purple line), and Non-Hispanic/Latinx White (solid green line) adults. For Non-Hispanic/Latinx White adults, the effect of male sex is significant from ages 22 to age 70, such that male individuals are at greater risk for hypertension than female individuals at these ages. For Non-Hispanic/Latinx Black adults, the effect of male sex is significant from ages 20 to 40 and ages 59 to 79, but the odds are <1.0, indicating that Non-Hispanic/Latinx Black males are at lesser risk for hypertension at these ages than Non-Hispanic/Latinx Black females. Lastly, the effect of male sex among Hispanic/Latinx adults is significant and >1.0 from ages 18 to 29 and 39 to 44 and significant and <1.0 from ages 57 to 77. Thus, male Hispanic/Latinx adults are at higher risk for hypertension in young and middle adulthood, but female Hispanic/Latinx adults are at higher risk in their late 50s through late 70s.

Differences can also be observed when comparing groups. As demonstrated by non-overlapping confidence intervals between the groups, the effect of male sex for Non-Hispanic/Latinx Black adults relative to Hispanic/Latinx adults is lower from approximately ages 18 to 40 and, relative to Non-Hispanic/Latinx White adults, the effect of male sex is lower from approximately ages 20 to 46 and again from ages 56 to 74. Differences were not as large when comparing Non-Hispanic/Latinx White and Hispanic/Latinx adults; small but significant differences were observed only between ages 31 and 43 and between ages 56 and 74 with the effect of male sex being stronger for Non-Hispanic/Latinx White adults relative to Hispanic/Latinx adults at those ages.

3.2 Part II. Generalized TVEM to Model Count Outcomes

Just as binary outcomes can be modeled with logistic TVEM, count outcomes can be modeled with Poisson TVEM. Some examples of count outcomes include the number of child abuse incidents in a month, the number of school students sent to a principal's office in a week, and the number of arrests made per day due to driving under the influence. Common features of the distribution of the outcome are that values cannot be negative—they must be whole numbers—and in theory, the mean and the variance of a Poisson distribution are equal (in practice, the variance often is larger than the mean, a condition referred to as overdispersion). Standard Poisson regression for count outcomes relies on the natural log transformation of the count outcome (i.e., response variable), Y.

Because the log of the expected count is modeled as a function of the covariates, all estimated Poisson regression coefficients are on the log scale. The general interpretation of the intercept coefficient is the log of the expected count on the response variable when all covariates are zero. When all covariates are centered, the interpretation is the log of the expected count for individuals with average levels on all covariates. The general interpretation of the coefficient corresponding to a covariate is the difference in the log of expected counts corresponding to a one-unit change in the covariate variable, holding constant all other covariates in the model. If a coefficient's 95% confidence interval does not contain the value 0, we reject the null hypothesis that the coefficient equals zero, given the other covariates in the model. In other words, when the confidence interval does not contain zero, we conclude that the covariate is significantly associated with the outcome. Because coefficients represent associations with the log of the expected count, coefficients are typically transformed to facilitate interpretation by exponentiating them. Exponentiated slopes in Poisson regression are interpreted as incidence rate ratios. (Note that an incidence rate conveys the number of events over a time period; thus, the terms "rate" and "count" can be used somewhat interchangeably.) For example, if a binary indicator of treatment (coded 1) vs. control group (coded 0) has a coefficient of $\beta = .4$, the incidence rate ratio corresponding to that covariate is $e^{.4} = 1.5$. This can be interpreted as follows: holding all other covariates constant, individuals in the treatment group are expected to have a rate on the response variable that is 1.5 times greater than individuals in the control group. For example, if the response variable were minutes of physical activity in a day, if individuals in each group are equivalent on all other covariates, those who receive an intervention to promote physical activity are expected to report 1.5 times more minutes of physical activity in a day than those in the control group.

Following standard Poisson regression for count outcomes, Poisson TVEM relies on the natural log transformation of the count outcome, Y, so that regression coefficients (intercepts and slopes) can be examined as continuous functions of time. Specifying a Poisson distribution assumes that the dependent variable is a count variable with possible values of 0, 1, 2, and so on with a Poisson distribution, and that a log-linear regression link function should be used. Intercept-only Poisson TVEM is used to estimate the log-mean count on the response variable across continuous time. The exponentiated intercept coefficient function provides the estimated mean count across time. Covariates can be included in Poisson TVEM to estimate the expected difference in the log of expected counts corresponding to a one-unit change in the covariate, holding constant all other covariates in the model, as a function of continuous time. We note that weighted analysis is not currently possible in Poisson TVEM because the software has no SAS procedure to call for analyzing survey data with count outcomes (whereas procedures SURVEYREG and SURVEYLOGISTIC do exist for continuous and binary outcomes, respectively). Additionally, TVEM for a zero-inflated Poisson outcome distribution has not been implemented in current SAS software; this represents an important area for future research. Next, we provide an empirical demonstration of Poisson TVEM, in which we model the mean typical number of drinks as a function of age.

3.2.1 Example: Mean Typical Number of Drinks and Associations With Sex and Racial/Ethnic Group Across Age

In this section, we walk through an empirical example modeling the typical number of drinks of alcohol on a typical occasion (in the past year) across age and the age-varying associations of sex, racial/ethnic group, and their interaction with typical number of drinks. Data are from NESARC-III (Grant et al., 2014), a nationally representative sample of more than 36,000 US adults aged 18 and older. Data from this cross-sectional study were collected in 2012 and 2013. We restricted our analytic dataset to individuals who were between the ages of 18 and 35 who did not report lifetime abstinence from alcohol use (n = 10,852). Within this restricted sample, 50.4% of participants were female. Regarding racial/ethnic group, 59.4% were Non-Hispanic/Latinx White, 20.3% were Hispanic/Latinx, 12.8% were Non-Hispanic/Latinx Black, 5.9% were Non-Hispanic Asian/Native Hawaiian/Other Pacific Islander, and 1.6% were Non-Hispanic American Indian/Alaskan Native.

The primary variables for this analysis included sex, typical number of drinks, and racial/ethnic group. Sex was coded as 1 = male and 0 = female. Typical number of drinks was coded as a count variable, with values ranging from 0 to 25 drinks (missing cases and typical number of drinks higher than 25 [n = 56] were excluded from analyses). We created dummy codes for racial/ethnic group, with Non-Hispanic/Latinx White adults as the reference group, including *BLACK* (1 = Non-Hispanic/Latinx Black, 0 = not Non-Hispanic/Latinx Black), *HISPANIC* (1 = Hispanic/Latinx, 0 = not Hispanic/Latinx), and *OTHER* (1 = Asian/Native Hawaiian/Other Pacific Islander or American Indian/Alaskan Native, 0 = not one of these groups).

For the purpose of this didactic example, we had three research questions:

Research Question 1: What is the age-varying mean number of drinks consumed on a typical drinking occasion in the past year, across ages 18–35?

Research Question 2: What are the age-varying differences in the mean typical number of drinks per drinking occasion consumed in the past year by sex and by racial/ethnic group?

Research Question 3: Is there an interaction between sex and racial/ethnic group in predicting mean typical number of drinks consumed per drinking occasion in the past year?

3.2.2 *Research Question 1: What is the Age-Varying Mean Number of Drinks Consumed on a Typical Drinking Occasion in the Past Year, Across Ages 18–35?*

An intercept-only TVEM was used to estimate the mean typical number of drinks (*TYPDRK2*) in the past year as a continuous function of age from 18 to 35 years. Let λ_i represent the mean number of drinks in a typical drinking occasion for individual i. Because λ is constrained to be nonnegative and the equal variance assumption in linear regression is violated for a count outcome, we apply the log-linear regression link function. The model is expressed as

$$ln(\lambda_i) = \beta_0(t),$$

where λ determines both the mean and variance of the count outcome (i.e., the Poisson variable), typical number of drinks. $\beta_0(t)$ is the coefficient function expressing the log of the mean (i.e., expected) typical number of drinks across continuous age. Values across age on this function can be exponentiated to facilitate interpretation; $e^{\beta_0(t)}$ is interpreted as the mean typical number of drinks across age. To estimate this model, we specified a %TVEM macro statement in SAS.

```
%TVEM(
data = nesarc_chapter3b,
dist = Poisson,
id = caseid,
time = nage,
dv = typdrk2,
tvary_effect = int,
method = P-spline,
knots = 10);
```

Because the outcome is a count variable, we specify the distribution to be "Poisson" in our **dist** statement. The **data** statement specifies the name of our working dataset. The **id** statement refers to our participant ID variable, *CASEID*; because this is a cross-sectional dataset, each row in our vertical dataset represents one participant's responses. **Time** refers to how we specify time on the *x*-axis; in this case, time is considered participants' age, denoted *NAGE*. **DV** is the outcome of interest; here, our outcome is the typical number of alcoholic drinks consumed on a drinking occasion during the past year, labeled as *TYPDRK2*. Because this simple model evaluates only the estimated mean of the dependent variable (*TYPDRK2*) across age, our **tvary_effect** specifies that only one coefficient function, for the intercept, will be estimated. We have already created a variable in our dataset (called *INT*) that is equal to 1 for all rows of data.

For this example, we specify the estimation **method** to be P-spline. Our **knots** statement refers to the number of splitting points we are specifying for our model, with a higher number of knots corresponding to the possibility of estimating a more complex coefficient function. As noted in Chap. 2, because our analysis uses P-spline estimation, model selection (i.e., selecting the most appropriate complexity of the coefficient functions) is done automatically. Because this simple model only estimates the intercept as a function of time, we only need to specify the number of knots for the intercept function.

A figure is automatically produced by the %TVEM macro showing how the intercept, as expressed by its estimated coefficient function $\beta_0(t)$, changes over time, along with corresponding 95% confidence intervals are also shown. Recall that the interpretation of the intercept in Poisson regression is in relation to the log-mean. Thus, for Poisson TVEM specifically, users are encouraged to exponentiate the intercept function and the corresponding confidence bands to plot $e^{\beta_0(t)}$, the estimated mean across age.

Several SAS datasets are automatically stored in the SAS Work directory. As noted in Chap. 2, the estimated coefficient functions are stored in the dataset **tvem_plot_data**. These datasets contain the information that was used to produce the figures shown in the SAS output. When specifying a Poisson outcome in logistic TVEM, odds ratios are not provided in the dataset; users must either (1) transform parameter estimates and confidence interval limits in SAS prior to exporting the file to Excel or (2) export the file to Excel and transform the parameter estimates in Excel prior to plotting. In our example, we first ran the %TVEM macro syntax for the intercept-only model shown above, then exported the SAS working dataset called **tvem_plot_data** into Excel as follows.

```
PROC EXPORT DATA=tvem_plot_data DBMS=xlsx
OUTFILE="C:\FolderName\typ_drinks.xlsx";
run;
```

Table 3.4 contains the first several rows of data that would be shown after opening the file in Excel. The variable *nage* is our indicator of time, representing participants' ages. Values range from 18 to 35, with 100 equal intervals across that age range. The variable *INT* represents the estimate of the intercept function at each respective age; in other words, this column provides the log-mean number of alcoholic drinks on a typical occasion at that age. Similarly, *INT_L* and *INT_U* represent the associated age-varying lower and upper bound of the 95% confidence intervals for the log-mean number of drinks, respectively. We created three new variables by exponentiating the intercept and confidence intervals at each age, which we labeled *EXP_INT*, *EXP_INT_L*, and *EXP_INT_U*. We created Fig. 3.7 by plotting these values along the *x*-axis of *NAGE*. Thus, Fig. 3.7 shows the estimated mean typical number of drinks, along with the corresponding 95% confidence interval, across ages 18–35. At age 18, the mean typical number of drinks is 2.7 (95% CI = 2.4–2.9).

Table 3.4 First several rows of data contained in the tvem_plot_data dataset

nage	int_L	int	int_U	int_SE
18.0000	0.89600	0.98616	1.07632	0.046000
18.1717	0.93043	1.01101	1.09160	0.041113
18.3434	0.96184	1.03416	1.10647	0.036894
18.5152	0.99032	1.05564	1.12095	0.033323
18.6869	1.01597	1.07550	1.13503	0.030372
18.8586	1.03892	1.09380	1.14868	0.028000
19.0303	1.05933	1.11059	1.16185	0.026152
19.2020	1.07739	1.12591	1.17444	0.024757
19.3737	1.09330	1.13982	1.18634	0.023734
19.5455	1.10728	1.15236	1.19744	0.023000
19.7172	1.11953	1.16358	1.20763	0.022473
19.8889	1.13024	1.17353	1.21681	0.022084
20.0606	1.13958	1.18226	1.22494	0.021775
20.2323	1.14768	1.18982	1.23196	0.021501

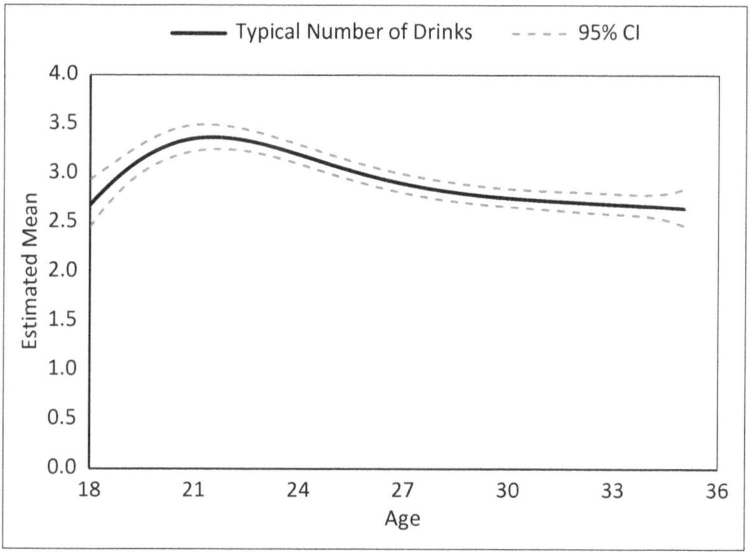

Fig. 3.7 Estimated mean number of alcoholic drinks consumed during a typical occasion in the past year as a function of age, derived by exponentiating the intercept function in logistic TVEM

There is an increase with age during very young adulthood, with the mean typical number of drinks peaking at age 21 with 3.4 drinks (CI = 3.2–3.5). The mean then gradually decreases with age to the minimum value of 2.6 (95% CI = 2.5–2.8) at age 35.

3.2.3 Research Question 2: What are the Age-Varying Differences in the Mean Typical Number of Drinks per Drinking Occasion Consumed in the Past Year by Sex and by Racial/Ethnic Group?

Next, covariates are added to estimate their age-varying effects on mean typical number of drinks. To facilitate exposition, sex and racial/ethnic group are examined in separate models.

3.2.3.1 Differences by Sex

We first estimate the effect of sex—indicated here with a variable named *MALE* (coded 1 = male, 0 = female)—on mean typical number of drinks across ages 18–35. The syntax, which allows for the association between sex and number of drinks to vary with age, is similar to that presented in Research Question 1, with two modifications.

```
%TVEM(
data = nesarc_chapter3b,
dist = Poisson,
id = caseid,
time = nage,
dv = typdrk2,
tvary_effect = int male,
method = P-spline,
knots = 10 10);
```

The first change is that we now add *MALE* as a covariate on the **tvary_effect** line of syntax in addition to the term for the intercept (*INT*). This will produce two age-varying coefficient functions, one for the intercept (interpreted as the log-mean typical number of drinks for female adults across age) and one for the coefficient of *MALE* (interpreted as the difference in log-mean typical number of drinks by sex). This specification allows the log-mean typical number of drinks to vary with age and allows the size of any sex difference also to vary with age. The second change is that we add a second specification for the number of **knots**, the first value for the intercept function and the second for the effect of *MALE*. As in Research Question 1, P-spline estimation is specified; thus, model selection (i.e., the level of complexity in each coefficient function across age) is handled automatically.

Running the TVEM macro syntax produces a coefficient function for the effect of *MALE*; however, unlike in logistic TVEM, in Poisson TVEM the program does not automatically calculate and plot the exponentiated coefficient function across age. This plot is important to create however to facilitate interpretation. The information needed to do so is stored in **tvem_plot_data**; by importing this dataset into Excel and exponentiating the coefficient function, the curve can then be interpreted as the incidence rate ratio for male individuals relative to female individuals. In Fig. 3.8a, we show the estimated coefficient function and associated 95%

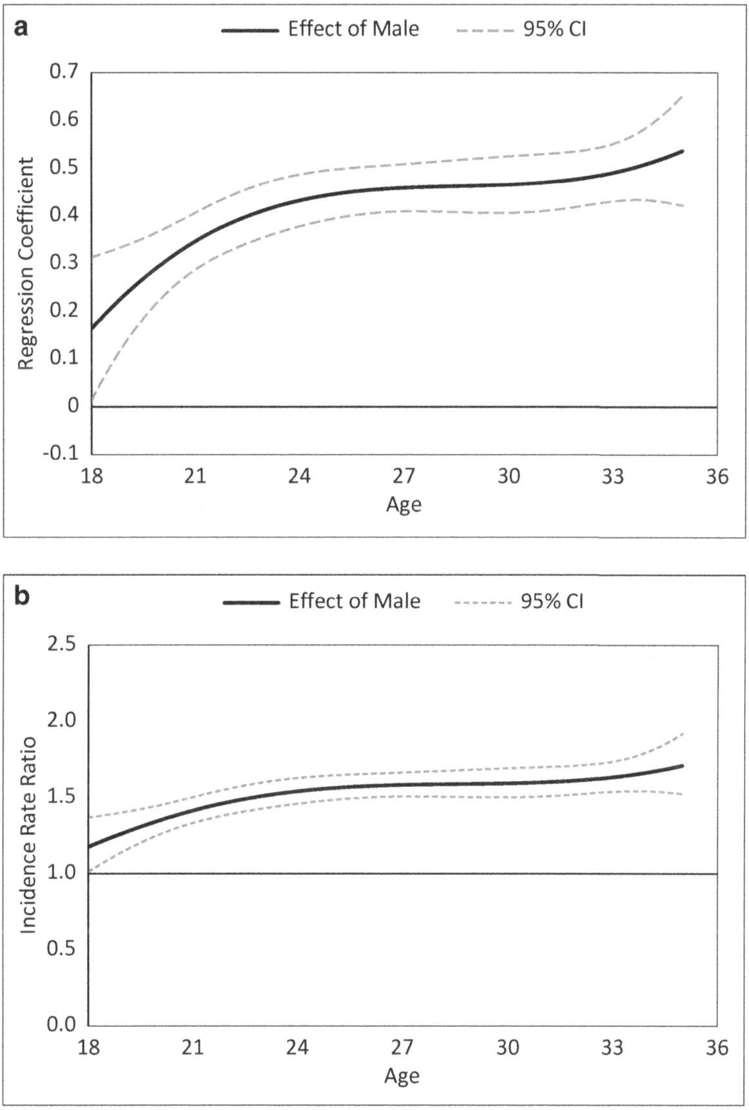

Fig. 3.8 (**a**) Age-dependent sex difference (i.e., the effect of being male) in the log-mean number of drinks consumed during a typical occasion across age. (An effect of 0 indicates no association.) (b) Incidence rate ratio representing age-dependent sex difference in the mean number of drinks consumed during a typical occasion across age. (An effect of 1 indicates no association.) (**c**) Estimated mean number of drinks consumed during a typical occasion across age separately for males and females

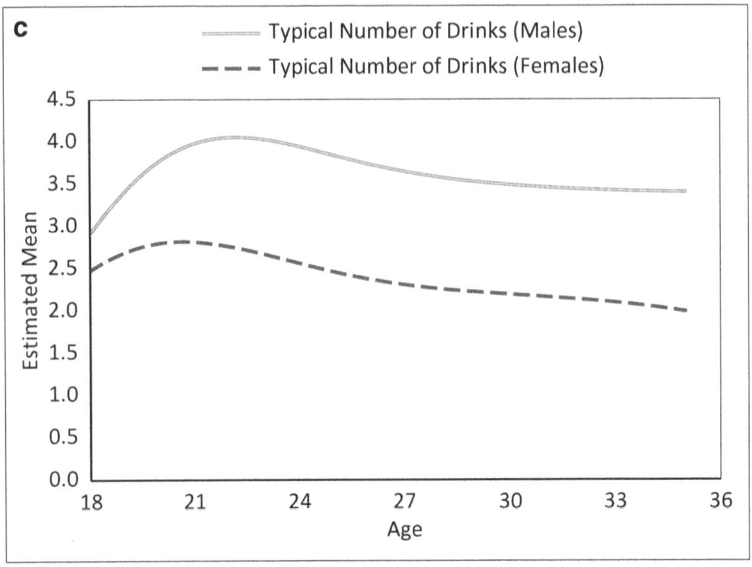

Fig. 3.8 (continued)

confidence interval for the effect of *MALE*; there is a statistically significant effect of sex for any ages at which the confidence interval does not include the value of 0; in this example, being male is associated with a significantly higher log-mean number of typical drinks compared to being female at all ages above 18. Figure 3.8b shows the same information, but we exponentiated the values shown in Fig. 3.8a so that we can interpret the curve as the age-varying incidence rate ratio. The solid black line represents the incidence rate ratio (IRR) associated with being male across age, and the dashed lines represent the associated 95% confidence band. The effect strengthens across age through around age 25 and then is quite stable across ages 25–35. At any given age, this effect indicates the multiplicative increase in the estimated mean typical number of drinks by sex. For example, at around age 23 the IRR equals 1.5, suggesting that at age 23, male adults are expected to have a number of typical drinks that is 1.5 times greater than female adults.

To further aid interpretation, we used the parameter estimates that had been imported into Excel to calculate the age-varying expected typical number of drinks by sex. Recall from Fig. 3.8a, b that the effect of sex was statistically significant across the entire age range; Fig. 3.8c aids in interpreting the effect size, how it changes with age, and the clinical significance of this finding across ages 18–35. Mean typical number of drinks among male adults (solid green line) is nearly 3 at age 18, rising to 4 drinks by age 21, then falling to 3.5 drinks in the 30s. The shape of the curve for female adults (dashed purple line) is similar, with a mean typical number of drinks of 2.5 at age 18 and peaking at about 2.8 drinks at age 21. Their curve however decreases with age into their 30s and is lowest at age 35, with a mean of 2 drinks.

3.2.3.2 Differences Across Racial/Ethnic Groups

We also tested differences across racial/ethnic group in the mean typical number of drinks across age. We examined the three largest groups in our dataset, Non-Hispanic/Latinx White, Non-Hispanic/Latinx Black, and Hispanic/Latinx adults, with remaining racial/ethnic categories combined into the Other group. Mean typical number of drinks was modeled as a function of main effects for racial/ethnic group using three dummy-coded indicators: *BLACK, HISPANIC, OTHER*. The following syntax was used to model the mean typical number of drinks across ages 18–35 as a function of racial/ethnic group, such that differences among racial/ethnic groups could vary across age.

```
%TVEM(
data = nesarc_chapter3b,
dist = Poisson,
id = caseid,
time = nage,
dv = typdrk2,
tvary_effect = int black hispanic other,
method = P-spline,
knots = 10 10 10 10);
```

Instead of including *MALE* as a covariate, we now specify *BLACK*, *HISPANIC*, and *OTHER* on the **tvary_effect** line of syntax, again in addition to the term for the intercept (*INT*). This will produce a total of four age-varying coefficient functions, one for the intercept (interpreted as the log-mean typical number of drinks for the reference group, Non-Hispanic/Latinx White adults, across age) and one each for the coefficients of *BLACK*, *HISPANIC*, and *OTHER* (each interpreted as the difference in the log-mean typical number of drinks for that racial/ethnic group compared to Non-Hispanic/Latinx White adults). This specification allows the log-mean typical number of drinks to vary with age and allows the size of any group difference also to vary with age. Because we are now estimating four coefficient functions, we must add two more specifications for the number of **knots**; these values correspond to the intercept function and the three coefficient functions representing the effect of racial/ethnic group (*BLACK*, *HISPANIC*, *OTHER*). The P-spline estimation procedure will automatically determine the level of complexity in each coefficient function across age.

Following a procedure similar to the one used to examine sex differences, we estimated the model by running the TVEM macro syntax. We then imported into

Excel the data stored in **tvem_plot_data** and exponentiated the coefficient functions for the three indicators of racial/ethnic group so that the curves could be more easily interpreted. These three IRR curves and associated 95% confidence bands are shown in Fig. 3.9a (note that, for brevity, we are not presenting a figure showing the pre-transformed coefficient functions because the IRR curves and corresponding confidence intervals convey the same information).

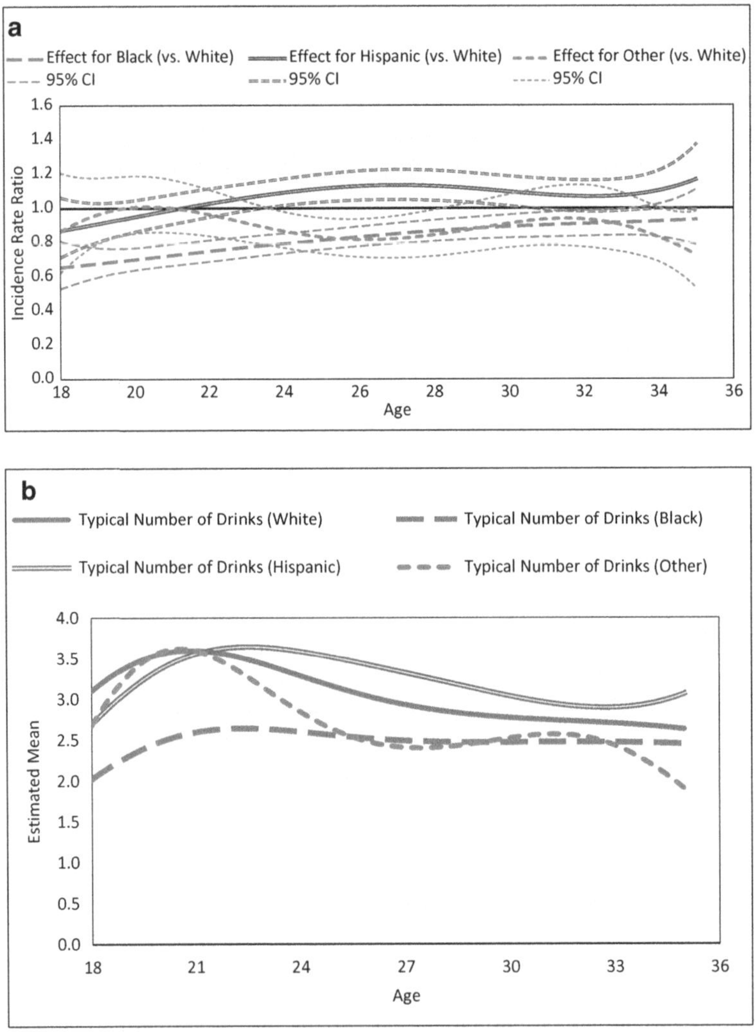

Fig. 3.9 (**a**) Incidence rate ratios representing the association between race/ethnicity and the mean number of drinks consumed during a typical occasion across age. (**b**) Estimated mean number of drinks consumed during a typical occasion across age for each racial/ethnic group

Racial/ethnic group and typical number of drinks are significantly associated in a somewhat complex way across the ages of 18 and 35. Figure 3.9a shows the age-varying IRRs and 95% confidence intervals corresponding to the associations between being in the Non-Hispanic/Latinx Black (long-dashed orange line), Hispanic/Latinx (double purple line), and Other (short-dashed blue line) groups compared to the Non-Hispanic/Latinx White group. Relative to Non-Hispanic/Latinx White adults, Non-Hispanic/Latinx Black adults have a significantly lower mean typical number of drinks from ages 18 to 34, whereas Hispanic/Latinx adults have a significantly higher mean typical number of drinks from ages 24 to 30. Results suggest that adults in the Other racial/ethnic group have a significantly lower mean typical number of drinks from ages 24 to 28, but additional research would be needed to confirm and better understand this finding given heterogeneity within the Other group. The strongest association was at age 18 when comparing Non-Hispanic/Latinx Black and White young adults. At this age the IRR equals less than 0.7, suggesting that Non-Hispanic/Latinx Black young adults are expected to have a number of typical drinks that is 0.7 times as high as Non-Hispanic/Latinx White young adults. To provide further context to these findings and to convey their clinical significance, the parameter estimates contained in **tvem_plot_data** were transformed to show the estimated typical number of drinks for each of the four racial/ethnic groups across age (see Fig. 3.9b). Indeed, the difference between mean typical number of drinks for Non-Hispanic/Latinx Black and White adults at age 18 stands out as one of the largest differences, with just 2 mean typical drinks for Non-Hispanic/Latinx Black adults at age 18 compared to more than 3 for Non-Hispanic/Latinx White adults at that age. The gap between these two groups lessens with age but remains statistically significant through about age 34 (per Fig. 3.9a).

3.2.4 Research Question 3: Is there an Interaction Between Sex and Racial/Ethnic Group in Predicting Mean Typical Number of Drinks Consumed per Drinking Occasion in the Past Year?

To answer the last research question, we tested the interaction of sex and racial/ethnic group in relation to mean typical number of drinks across age. This hierarchical model includes terms for the intercept (*INT*), the main effect of sex (*MALE*; female specified as the reference group), the main effects for racial/ethnic group (*BLACK, HISPANIC, OTHER*; Non-Hispanic/Latinx White adults specified as the reference group), and a set of interaction terms we created as the product of our sex and racial/ethnic group indicators (*SEXBLACK, SEXHISP, SEXOTHER*). Each of these variable names will be listed under the **tvary_effect** argument to allow any moderation effect (i.e., any sex by racial/ethnic group interaction) to vary flexibly across age.

```
%TVEM(
data = nesarc_chapter3b,
dist = Poisson,
id = caseid,
time = nage,
dv = typdrk2,
tvary_effect = int male black hispanic other
sexblack    sexhisp sexother,
method = P-spline,
knots = 10 10 10 10 10 10 10 10);
```

As with any TVEM specification, one value indicating the number of knots is specified for each time-varying effect. The coefficient functions of specific interest here, which allow us to test for significant moderation, are the coefficient functions for *SEXBLACK*, *SEXHISP*, and *SEXOTHER*, found in the **tvem_plot_data** working dataset.[4] These plots, shown in Fig. 3.10, represent the time-varying effect of the interaction of sex and racial/ethnic group in predicting the log-mean typical number of drinks across age. Any age at which the confidence intervals do not include the value of 0 indicate a significant moderation effect. As shown in Fig. 3.10a, a significant interaction effect was detected for Non-Hispanic/Latinx Black adults versus the reference group, Non-Hispanic/Latinx White adults, between approximately ages 25 and 30. Because the coefficient is significant and negative during those ages, we can interpret this as a smaller sex difference (i.e., a weaker effect of the covariate *MALE*) among Non-Hispanic/Latinx Black adults compared to the reference group. For Hispanic/Latinx adults, there is no significant difference in the effect of sex relative to the reference group at any age (Fig. 3.10b). A significant interaction effect emerged for adults in other racial/ethnic groups versus the reference group between approximately ages 22 and 26. The coefficient is significant and negative during those ages thus we can interpret this as a weaker sex difference among adults in other racial/ethnic groups compared to the reference group.

Had none of the interaction coefficient functions been significant at any age, we would conclude from the null result that there was no evidence for sex differences in mean typical drinks at any age, for any racial/ethnic group compared to the reference group, Non-Hispanic/Latinx White adults. In this case, we would not probe the interaction effect further and would report a main-effects model as a final model. However, in our case, we identified two significant interaction effects, one for Non-Hispanic/Latinx Black compared to the reference group and one for Others compared the reference group (see Fig. 3.10a, c). Next, we unpack these interaction effects to facilitate their interpretation.

One way to approach this interpretation would be to plot the effect of one variable (e.g., the effect of being male) across levels of the other variable (e.g., for each racial/ethnic group). In the hypertension example shown above, weighted TVEM was used for estimation; this allows use of the convenient **domain** and **which**

[4] When testing interactions, the β coefficient curve (prior to exponentiating) should be used instead of the incidence rate ratio curve, as this curve is not easily interpreted.

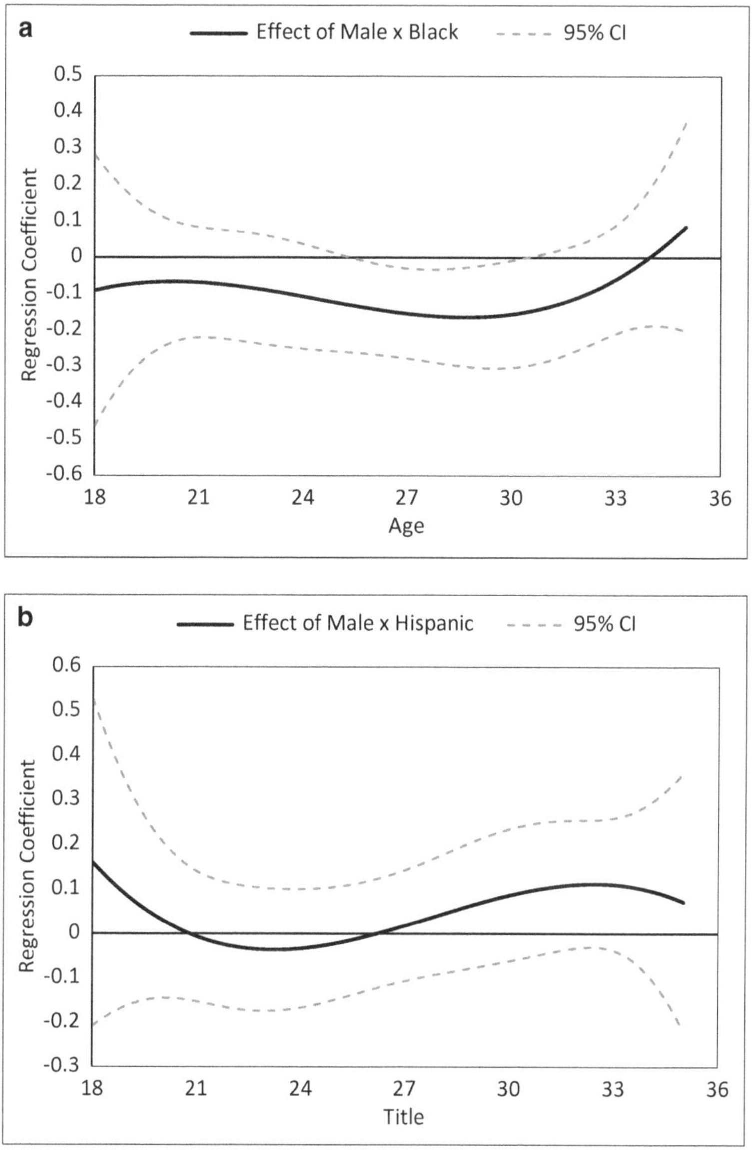

Fig. 3.10 Coefficient functions corresponding to the interaction between the indicator of being male and indicators of being (**a**) Black, (**b**) Hispanic/Latinx, and (**c**) Other racial/ethnic group on mean number of drinks during a typical occasion across age

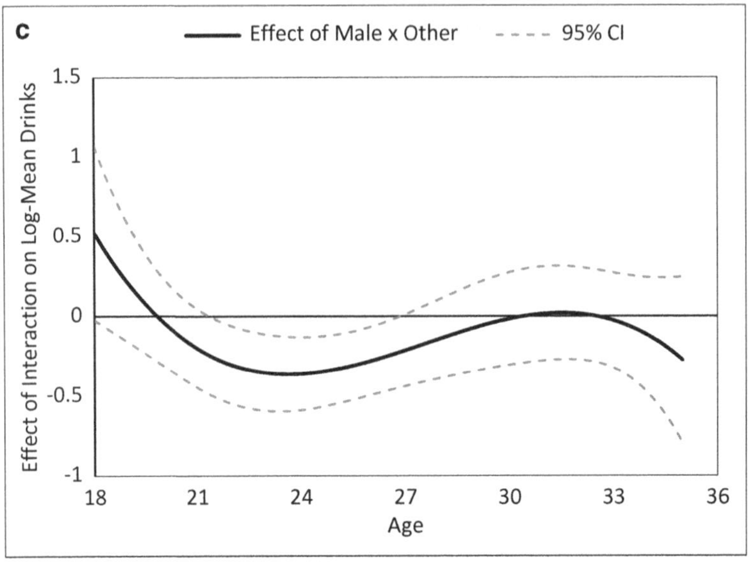

Fig. 3.10 (continued)

statements. With Poisson TVEM, weighted TVEM is not possible. Thus, to probe a time-varying interaction term predicting a count outcome, we recommend using one of two options. Let us consider racial/ethnic group to be the moderator variable and we wish to examine the effect of sex within each racial/ethnic group. In the first option, one could simply subset the data by levels of the moderator, for example, dividing the data into four smaller datasets based on racial/ethnic group. Then, the main effect of sex could be estimated in each dataset and results plotted on the same figure to facilitate comparison across groups. Second, one could run the same interaction model—including terms for the intercept, all main effects, and all interaction terms—several times, each time re-specifying the reference group on the moderator (i.e., re-centering the moderator variable). Our original model specification was based on coding racial/ethnic group so that the reference group is Non-Hispanic/Latinx White adults. In this specification, the main effect of being male is interpreted as the age-varying effect of sex for the reference group (those with a value of 0 on the set of indicators of racial/ethnic group, *BLACK*, *HISPANIC*, and *OTHER*). The second model would be identical, except that it could be based on racial/ethnic group coded such that, say, Non-Hispanic/Latinx Black adults are the reference group (i.e., indicators of racial/ethnic group would include dummy-coded variables *WHITE*, *HISPANIC*, and *OTHER*). For this re-specified model, the main effect of male now is interpreted as the age-varying effect of sex for Non-Hispanic/Latinx Black adults (again, those with a value of 0 on the set of indicators of racial/ethnic group). The model could be re-specified and re-estimated two more times, with Hispanic/Latinx adults and Other adults, respectively, coded as the reference group. The four group-specific coefficient functions for sex represent simple slopes and can be plotted together to facilitate comparison across groups.

Another way to facilitate interpretation, which we demonstrate here, is to calculate from the interaction model the estimated mean typical number of drinks across age for all sex-racial/ethnic subgroups. This is easily done in Excel using the parameter estimates that were imported from the **tvem_plot_data** file, and an example is included in the companion website for this book (https://prevention.psu.edu/books/tvem/). For example, the exponentiated intercept function from our interaction model represents the mean number of drinks during a typical occasion across age for female Non-Hispanic/Latinx White individuals (the reference group on both sex and racial/ethnic group). Similarly, exponentiating the sum of the intercept coefficient and the main effect of male yields the mean typical number of drinks for male Non-Hispanic/Latinx White individuals. This procedure works for calculating the estimated mean typical number of drinks for each sex-racial/ethnic group: at each value of age, we sum the coefficients relevant for that group (based on that group's coding on all of the dummy variable indicators) and exponentiate that value to calculate the estimated mean for that group. Figure 3.11 depicts the mean typical drinks for all eight sex-racial/ethnic groups across ages 18–35.

Recall from Fig. 3.10 that there were two age periods where significant moderation was found, at least when comparing Non-Hispanic/Latinx White adults to those in other racial/ethnic groups. The sex difference (i.e., the effect of the covariate *MALE*) at ages 25–30 was significantly different between the Non-Hispanic/Latinx Black and Non-Hispanic/Latinx White groups, as denoted by the brace and single asterisk on Fig. 3.11. Additionally, the effect of sex at ages 22–26 was significantly different between the Other and Non-Hispanic/Latinx White groups, as denoted by the brace and double asterisk. These particular interaction effects may be difficult to interpret as they are quite small, but the results in Fig. 3.10

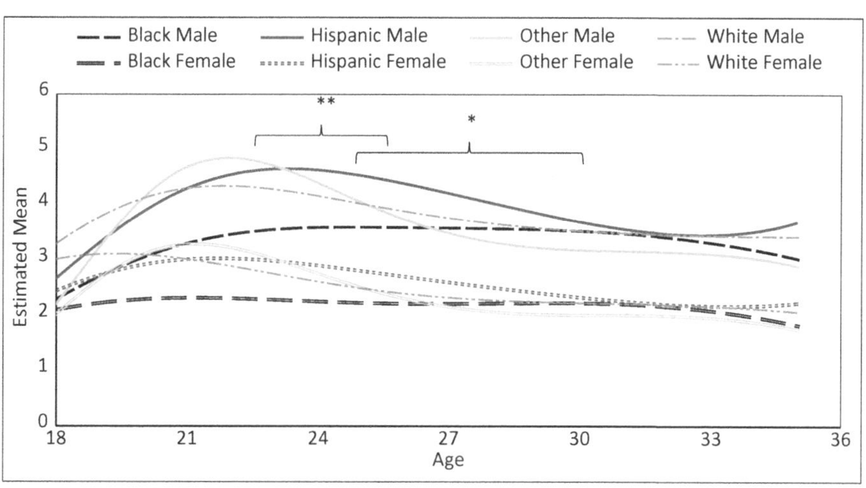

Fig. 3.11 Mean number of drinks during a typical occasion across age for sex and racial/ethnic groups. As indicated by braces, significant differences in the effect of sex were identified *between Black and White adults at ages 25–30 (see Fig. 3.9a), and **between Other and White adults at ages 22–26 (see Fig. 3.9c)

suggest that the relative difference in mean typical drinks among male compared to female adults may be slightly larger among Non-Hispanic/Latinx White adults than those in the Other racial/ethnic group between ages 22 and 26. Further research would be needed to confirm and explain this difference. One benefit of creating a plot such as Fig. 3.11 is that the clinical significance and relative strength of any differences can easily be determined by the reader. One can readily pick up from this figure the relative importance of sex differences, racial/ethnic group differences, and their interaction.

3.2.5 Sample Results Section

Sample Results Section: Mean Typical Number of Drinks

Research Question 1. Figure 3.7 shows the estimated mean typical number of drinks consumed, along with the corresponding 95% confidence interval (CI), across ages 18–35. At age 18, the mean typical number of drinks is 2.7 (95% CI = 2.4–2.9). There is an increase with age during very young adulthood, with the mean typical number of drinks peaking at age 21 with 3.6 drinks (CI = 3.2–3.5). The mean then gradually decreases with age to the minimum value of 2.6 (95% CI = 2.5–2.8) at age 35.

Research Question 2. Figure 3.8b shows the exponentiated coefficient function for the effect of being male; this is interpreted as the age-varying incidence rate ratio (IRR). The solid black line represents the IRR associated with being male across age, and the dashed lines represent the associated 95% CI across age. The effect is significant across all ages; it strengthens across age through around age 25 and then is quite stable across ages 25–35. At any given age, this effect indicates the multiplicative increase in the estimated mean typical number of drinks for male adults compared to female adults. For example, at around age 23 the IRR equals 1.5, suggesting that at age 23, male adults are expected to have a number of typical drinks that is 1.5 times greater compared to female adults.

To further aid interpretation, the coefficient functions were used to calculate the expected typical number of drinks across age by sex. Figure 3.8c show that among male adults, the mean typical number of drinks is nearly 3 at age 18, rising to 4 drinks by age 21, then falling to 3.5 drinks in their 30s. The shape of the curve for female adults is similar, with a mean typical number of drinks of 2.5 at age 18 and peaking at about 2.8 drinks at age 21. The curve for female adults however decreases with age into their 30s and is lowest at age 35 with a mean of just 2 drinks.

Racial/ethnic group and typical number of drinks are significantly associated in a somewhat complex way across ages 18–35. Figure 3.9a shows the age-varying IRRs and 95% CIs corresponding to the associations between being a Non-Hispanic/Latinx Black, Hispanic/Latinx, or Other adult compared to being a Non-Hispanic/Latinx White adult. Relative to Non-Hispanic/Latinx White adults, Non-Hispanic/Latinx Black adults have a significantly lower mean typical number of drinks from ages 18 to 34, and Other adults have a significantly lower mean typical number of drinks from ages 24 to 28, whereas Hispanic/Latinx adults have a significantly higher mean typical number of drinks from ages 24 to 30. The strongest association was at age 18, between Non-Hispanic/Latinx Black and Non-Hispanic/Latinx White adults. At this age the IRR equals less than 0.7, suggesting that Non-Hispanic/Latinx Black adults are expected to have a number of typical drinks that is 0.7 times as high as Non-Hispanic/Latinx White adults. To provide further context, the parameter estimates were transformed to show the estimated typical number of drinks for each of the four racial/ethnic groups across age (see Fig. 3.9b). Indeed, the difference between mean typical number of drinks for Non-Hispanic/Latinx Black and Non-Hispanic/Latinx White adults at age 18 stands out as the widest gap, with just 2 mean typical drinks for Non-Hispanic/Latinx Black adults at age 18 compared to more than 3 for Non-Hispanic/Latinx White adults at that age. The gap between these two groups lessens with age but remains statistically significant through about age 34 (per Fig. 3.9a).

Research Question 3. In addition to exploring the main effects of sex and race-ethnicity on mean typical number of drinks as a function of continuous age, we specified a moderation model to examine whether sex and race-ethnicity interact in predicting mean typical number of drinks across age. Specifically, we examined whether sex differences across age in the mean typical number of drinks differed for Non-Hispanic/Latinx White individuals, compared to Non-Hispanic/Latinx Black individuals and Hispanic/Latinx individuals. As shown in Fig. 3.10, a significant interaction effect emerged for Non-Hispanic/Latinx Black adults versus the reference group, Non-Hispanic/Latinx White adults, between approximately ages 25 and 30. Because the coefficient is significant and negative during those ages, we can interpret this as a weaker effect of being male among Non-Hispanic/Latinx Black adults compared to Non-Hispanic/Latinx White adults. For Hispanic/Latinx adults, there is no significant difference in the effect of sex relative to Non-Hispanic/Latinx White adults at any age. A significant interaction effect emerged for adults in other racial/ethnic groups versus the reference group, Non-Hispanic/Latinx White adults, between approximately ages 22 and 26. The coefficient is significant and negative during those ages thus we can interpret this as a weaker effect of being male among adults in other racial/ethnic groups compared to Non-Hispanic/Latinx White adults. To facilitate the interpretation of effects in this complex model, Fig. 3.11 presents the mean number of drinks during a typical occasion for each sex-racial/ethnic group across ages 18–35.

References

Agresti, A. (2015). *Foundations of linear and generalized linear models*. John Wiley & Sons.

Grant, B. F., Chu, A., Sigman, R., Amsbary, M., Kali, J., Sugawara, Y., Jiao, R., Ren, W., & Goldstein, R. (2014). *Source and accuracy statement: National Epidemiologic Survey on Alcohol and Related Conditions-III (NESARC-III)* (pp. 1–125). National Institute on Alcohol Abuse and Alcoholism.

Vasilenko, S. A., Piper, M. E., Lanza, S. T., Liu, X., Yang, J., & Li, R. (2014). Time-varying processes involved in smoking lapse in a randomized trial of smoking cessation therapies. *Nicotine & Tobacco Research, 16*(Suppl_2), S135–S143.

Chapter 4
Time-Varying Effect Modeling to Study Age-Varying Associations

4.1 Examining Differences in Associations Across Age Using TVEM

Although it was originally developed to model changes across time using intensive longitudinal data, time-varying effect modeling (TVEM) has increasingly been applied to examine changes across age using cross-sectional and longitudinal data-sets. Modeling changes in the mean level (or the prevalence) of an outcome as a function of continuous age or modeling the association between two variables across age can elucidate epidemiological or developmental patterns. Traditionally, examining change in a construct across age involves the use of regression analysis, including growth curve modeling. Methods for analyzing how outcomes vary across age typically assume that the effects of the covariates in an analysis are static. For example, even though something like the impact of perceptions of peer approval on mental health outcomes may differ from adolescence to older adulthood, in a traditional linear regression this time-varying association is not taken into account. TVEM allows scientists to flexibly model this type of time-varying association.

TVEM can be used to model age trends in repeated measures or cross-sectional data. For example, Flannery, Vannucci, and Ohannessian (2018) used TVEM to model developmental changes in coping strategies by combining two samples: (a) adolescents followed longitudinally across 4 years of high school and 5 years post-graduation and (b) a nationally representative cross-sectional study of 18–22-year-olds. Prior work examining coping strategies typically examined results across different age groups (e.g., 9–12, 13–15, 16–19, 20–29; Amirkhan & Auyeung, 2007). The flexibility of TVEM for modeling nonparametric associations across age allowed Flannery and colleagues to detect key changes in adolescents' and young adults' use of coping strategies (i.e., active coping, social support seeking, planning, venting emotions) across the transition from adolescence into young adulthood. These researchers also identified significant differences by age for male individuals

S. T. Lanza, A. N. Linden-Carmichael, *Time-Varying Effect Modeling for the Behavioral, Social, and Health Sciences*,
https://doi.org/10.1007/978-3-030-70944-0_4

compared to female individuals. Detecting fluctuations in coping strategies across developmental time, as well as in age-varying sex differences, offers key insights for advancing prevention and intervention programs tailored to certain ages. Such fine-grained, age-varying changes would not otherwise have been detected if individuals were compared by collapsing across age into coarse age groups.

Another published example used cross-sectional data to examine the prevalence of an emerging public health concern, *high-intensity drinking*, or the consumption of 8+/10+ drinks in one sitting for females/males and the association between high-intensity drinking and a past-year alcohol use disorder (Linden-Carmichael, Vasilenko, Lanza, & Maggs, 2017). Using data from a subset of participants in the National Epidemiologic Survey on Alcohol and Related Conditions-III (NESARC-III; Grant et al., 2014), researchers used TVEM to estimate the prevalence of high-intensity drinking relative to lower, yet still risky levels of drinking ("binge drinking") across ages 18–64. Further, researchers modeled the relative odds of experiencing an alcohol use disorder for high-intensity drinkers relative to binge-only drinkers. Findings demonstrated that across all ages, high-intensity drinkers were at greater odds of experiencing a recent use disorder, but that this association was strongest for young adults. Similar to longitudinal findings from Flannery et al. (2018), these findings highlight the importance of prevention and intervention at key ages.

4.1.1 Research Questions

This chapter presents an example using the same data as in Linden-Carmichael et al. (2017). In this chapter, we also consider the age-varying prevalence and comorbidity of the two most common mental health disorders in the United States (Moffitt et al., 2007), generalized anxiety disorder (GAD) and major depressive disorder (MDD), as well as age-varying changes in prevalence and comorbidity by sex. We walk the reader through the analytic dataset, statistical models specified to address each research question, and careful interpretation of each result. We provide SAS syntax and equations for each model in the online Appendix on the companion website (https://prevention.psu.edu/books/tvem/). Specifically, we address four research questions.

Research Question 1: What are the estimated prevalence rates of past-year GAD and past-year MDD across ages 18–65?

Research Question 2: How does the association between past-year MDD and past-year GAD change across continuous age?

Research Question 3: How does the association between sex and GAD change across continuous age?

Research Question 4: How does sex moderate, across age, the association between past-year GAD and past-year MDD? (In other words, how does the sex difference in the association between GAD and MDD differ across age?)

4.2 Method

4.2.1 Sample

Data were from NESARC-III, a large, nationally representative sample of 36,309 noninstitutionalized US adults aged 18 and older. Data were collected in 2012 and 2013. Black, Hispanic/Latinx, and Asian adults were oversampled to provide more reliable estimates. In the present analysis, we restricted our sample to individuals aged 18–65 (due to relative sparseness of data among adults older than 65 years), yielding an analytic sample of 30,999 adults (51.1% female).

4.2.2 Measures

The Alcohol Use Disorder and Associated Disabilities Interview Schedule (AUDADIS-5; Grant et al., 2011), a structured diagnostic interview developed by the National Institute on Alcohol Abuse and Alcoholism, was used to measure selected mood, anxiety, and substance use disorders. The AUDADIS-5 has demonstrated good validity and reliability (Grant et al., 2015; Hasin et al., 2015). In accordance with the Diagnostic and Statistical Manual of Mental Disorders (DSM-5; American Psychiatric Association, 2013), individuals were coded based on whether they met criteria for *GAD* during the past year (coded 1 = yes, during the past 12 months, 0 = no, not during the past 12 months). Similarly, individuals were coded based on whether they met criteria for *MDD* during the past year (coded 1 = yes, during the past 12 months, 0 = no, not during the past 12 months). *SEX* was coded as 1 = male and 0 = female. There were no missing data on any study variables.

4.2.3 Statistical Analysis

Estimates for all descriptive statistics and models were weighted to ensure a better representation of adults in the US. We specified a series of weighted logistic time-varying effect models to estimate regression coefficients as a function of cross-sectional age. The companion website for this book (https://prevention.psu.edu/books/tvem/) shows the statistical model and syntax used to specify each time-varying effect model used to address the research questions in this study; model numbers used below correspond to those on the website to aid the reader. Coefficients in logistic TVEM are automatically transformed (i.e., exponentiated) to show corresponding odds ratios (ORs), but given our interest in displaying estimated prevalence rates for the sample and prevalence rates across levels of covariates, we manually transformed the coefficient functions to reflect prevalence rates for the purpose of plotting results. These transformations are documented in the Appendix on the companion website (https://prevention.psu.edu/books/tvem/). A detailed overview of how to conduct logistic TVEM is provided in Chap. 3.

To address Research Question 1 (the estimated prevalence of past-year GAD and past-year MDD across ages 18–65), we separately conducted intercept-only logistic TVEM to estimate the prevalence of past-year GAD and the prevalence of past-year MDD across ages 18–65 (Models 4.1 and 4.2, respectively). Specifically, Model 4.1 estimated an intercept-only model for the odds of past-year GAD as a nonparametric function of continuous age, and Model 4.2 estimated an intercept-only model for the odds of past-year MDD across continuous age. Logistic TVEM output produces the intercept regression coefficient function and the corresponding odds across age. We transformed these odds to reflect estimated prevalence rates across age for both Models 4.1 and 4.2.

To answer Research Question 2 (the association between past-year MDD and past-year GAD across age), we used logistic TVEM to model past-year MDD as an age-varying covariate predicting past-year GAD (Model 4.3).

For Research Question 3 (the association between sex and GAD across age), logistic TVEM was used to model sex as a covariate predicting of past-year GAD (Model 4.4). Although sex is a time-invariant variable, we specified it to have a time-varying effect to allow us to examine how sex is associated with GAD across ages 18–65. As the indicator of sex was coded 1 for male and 0 for female, findings can be interpreted as the differences between males and females in the log-odds of past-year GAD.

Lastly, to test Research Question 4 (sex as a moderator of the association between past-year GAD and past-year MDD across age), we modeled past-year GAD as a function of MDD, sex, and their interaction, each specified as having age-varying effects (Model 4.5). To interpret the interaction and further examine the association between past-year GAD and MDD by sex, we also estimated the association between GAD and MDD for male and female adults separately (Models 4.6a and 4.6b, respectively). Models 4.6a and 4.6b included the intercept and past-year MDD as time-varying covariates, and analyses were conducted separately with an indicator of sex specified in the **domain** statement (see Chaps. 2 and 3 for more information on using a **domain** statement). As shown in the syntax provided in the Appendix on the companion website (https://prevention.psu.edu/books/tvem/), in Model 4.6a, the **domain** statement is specified to be "1" to estimate the age-varying association between MDD and GAD among males, and in Model 4.6b, the **domain** statement is specified to be "0" to estimate this association among females. Results for males and females were plotted together to facilitate interpretation of sex differences across age.

Because certain groups were oversampled in NESARC-III, all descriptive statistics and analyses were weighted. Thus, B-spline was used in all models, requiring model selection to be conducted manually. The most appropriate number of knots was selected for each model by comparing AIC and BIC for models with different numbers of knots for each covariate. The most appropriate number of knots selected for each model is presented in syntax found in the Appendix. Details concerning the use of sample weights and selecting the optimal number of knots with B-spline estimation are described in Chap. 2.

4.3 Results

4.3.1 Research Question 1: What are the Estimated Prevalence Rates of Past-Year Generalized Anxiety Disorder and Past-Year Major Depressive Disorder Across Ages 18–65?

The weighted estimate of the prevalence of past-year GAD across the entire sample was 5.6% and the past-year prevalence of MDD was 11.4%. Two intercept-only logistic time-varying effect models were specified to address this research question, one with GAD as the outcome and one with MDD. For both, the intercept coefficient was specified to be time-varying. The estimated prevalence of past-year GAD as a function of continuous age is presented in Fig. 4.1 with corresponding 95% confidence intervals. As in standard logistic regression, at any given age, t, the estimated prevalence can be calculated by exponentiating the coefficient function, $\beta_0(t)$, and dividing by 1 plus the exponentiated coefficient function at each time, as follows:

$$P(t) = \frac{e^{\beta_0(t)}}{1 + e^{\beta_0(t)}}.$$

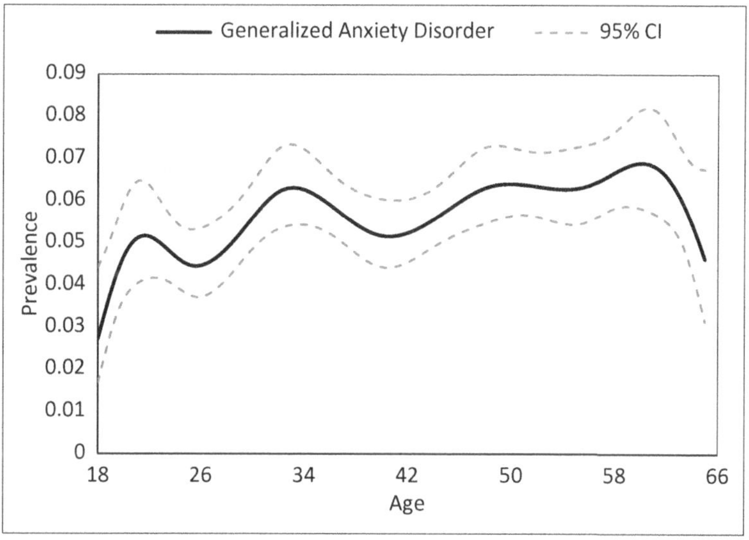

Fig. 4.1 Estimated prevalence (with 95% confidence band) of past-year generalized anxiety disorder as a function of continuous age

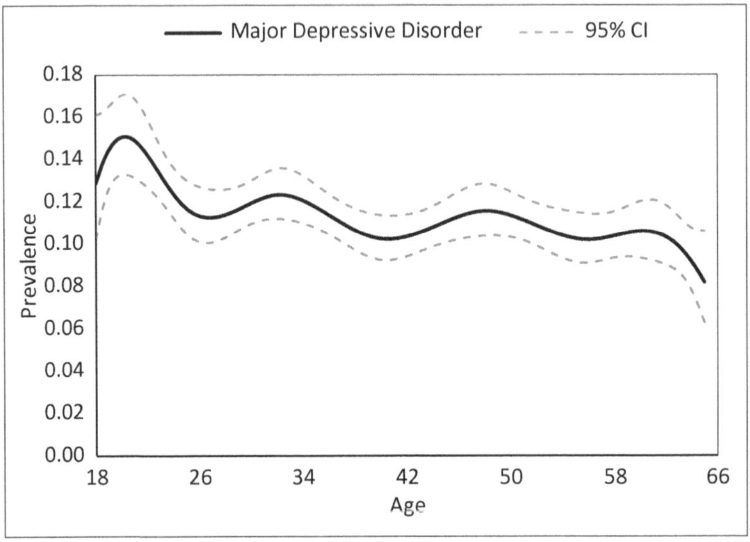

Fig. 4.2 Estimated prevalence (with 95% confidence band) of past-year major depressive disorder as a function of continuous age

Although estimates were somewhat "wiggly" across age, prevalence rates were generally stable across ages 18–65, ranging from a minimum of 2.7% at age 18 to a maximum of 6.9% at age 60, with the prevalence steadily declining with age for adults over age 60. Results were derived from Model 4.1 (see Appendix for details on model specification and selection and the corresponding syntax).

Figure 4.2 shows the age-varying prevalence of past-year MDD with corresponding 95% confidence intervals. The prevalence of past-year MDD showed a somewhat steady decline across age. Prevalence peaked among adults around age 20, with 15.1% of individuals at this age reporting past-year MDD. Rates were lowest among adults age 65, with 8.2% reporting past-year MDD. Results were derived from Model 4.2 (see Appendix for the corresponding syntax).

4.3.2 *Research Question 2: How Does the Association Between Past-Year MDD and Past-Year GAD Change Across Continuous Age?*

To address this research question, a logistic TVEM was specified with log-odds of GAD as the outcome and MDD as a covariate specified to have an age-varying coefficient:

$$ln\left(\frac{P(GAD)}{1+P(GAD)}\right)=\beta_0(t)+\beta_1(t)MDD_i.$$

Figure 4.3 shows the estimated association between past-year MDD as a covariate of past-year GAD. Specifically, this TVEM compares the relative odds of experiencing past-year GAD for individuals who also experienced MDD in the past year relative to individuals who did not experience past-year MDD. Findings demonstrate that, across all ages, past-year MDD is positively associated with odds of having past-year GAD. The significance of this finding is demonstrated by confidence intervals (dashed lines) that do not include the value of 1 (indicated on the figure by a horizontal line). This association between MDD and GAD is positive and strengthens fairly linearly across age, such that the association between MDD and GAD is lowest at age 18 (OR = 3.75) and highest at age 60 (OR = 9.06). In other words, although meeting criteria for MDD during the past year is strongly and positively associated with GAD at all ages, the increased odds of GAD associated with MDD is nearly three times higher among older adults. These results were based on Model 4.3, specified above (see Appendix for the corresponding syntax).

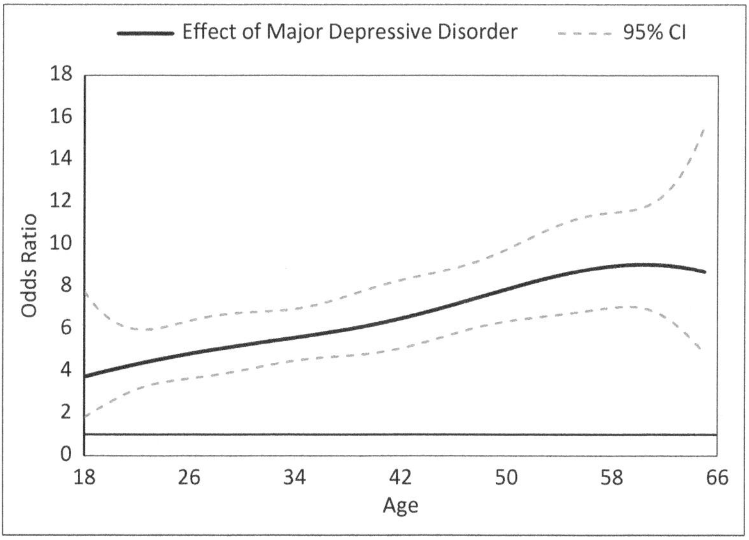

Fig. 4.3 Estimated change in odds of meeting criteria for a past-year generalized anxiety disorder (with 95% confidence band) associated with having a past-year major depressive disorder as a function of age

4.3.3 Research Question 3: How Does the Association Between Sex and GAD Change Across Continuous Age?

Similar to addressing Research Question 2, Model 4.4 tests the age-varying association between sex and past-year GAD:

$$ln\left(\frac{P(GAD)}{1+P(GAD)}\right)=\beta_0(t)+\beta_1(t)SEX_i.$$

As shown in Fig. 4.4, because the confidence intervals do not include the value 1.0 at any age, there are significant differences by sex in the odds of having a past-year GAD across ages 18–65. As *SEX* is coded 1 for male and 0 for female, the age-specific association can be interpreted as the effect of being male (relative to female) on past-year GAD. Further, odds ratios are less than 1.0 at each age, indicating that male individuals exhibit significantly lower odds of having a past-year GAD across age than female individuals. The association between sex and GAD is strongest at age 18, with an OR of 0.30; at age 18, male adults are 30% as likely as female adults to report GAD. This association weakens from ages 18–29, with the weakest effect at approximately age 29 with an OR of 0.71 (recall that an OR of 1.0 indicates no association). For adults older than 29, this association steadily declines with age until approximately age 46, with male adults about half as likely as female adults to report GAD across ages 46–65. These results were based on Model 4.4, which is specified above (see Appendix for the corresponding syntax).

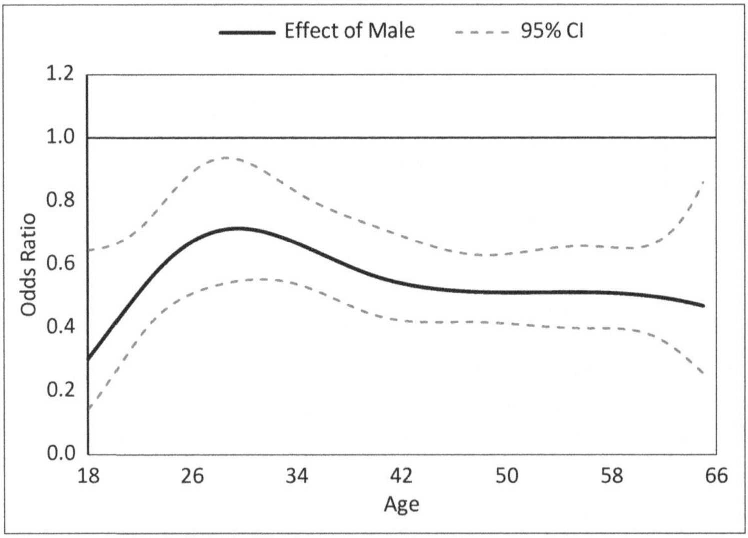

Fig. 4.4 Estimated change in odds of meeting criteria for a past-year generalized anxiety disorder (with 95% confidence band) associated with being male as a function of age

4.3.4 Research Question 4: How Does Sex Moderate, Across Age, the Association Between Past-Year GAD and Past-Year MDD? (In Other Words, How Does the Sex Difference in the Association Between GAD and MDD Differ Across Age?)

Our final model examined the interaction effect of past-year MDD and sex on the odds of past-year GAD across ages 18–65. As shown in Model 4.5, we first created an interaction term of past-year MDD by sex. To test this interaction, we included the intercept, past-year MDD, sex, and the interaction term as covariates of past-year GAD; all were specified to have age-varying effects. This model was specified as

$$ln\left(\frac{P(GAD)}{1+P(GAD)}\right) = \beta_0(t) + \beta_1(t)MDD_i + \beta_2(t)SEX_i + \beta_3(t)MDD_iSEX_i.$$

The coefficient functions $\beta_1(t)$ and $\beta_2(t)$ express the time-varying main effects of past-year MDD and sex, respectively. Given the dummy variable coding of MDD_i and SEX_i, $\beta_1(t)$ represents the age-varying association between MDD and GAD for female individuals (where $SEX_i = 0$), and $\beta_2(t)$ represents the age-varying association between sex and GAD among those who did not meet criteria for MDD in the past year (where $MDD_i = 0$). Figure 4.5 shows the interaction term of MDD by sex,

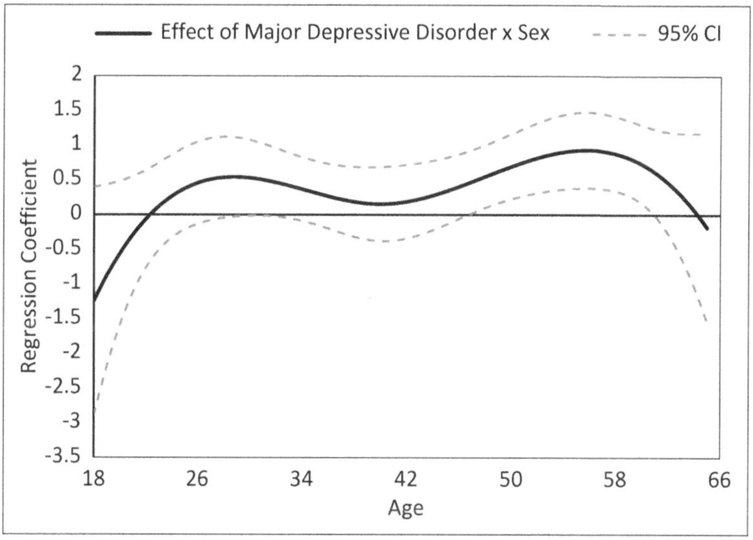

Fig. 4.5 Age-varying effect of the interaction between past-year major depressive disorder and sex predicting past-year generalized anxiety disorder as a function of age. Ages at which confidence intervals do not include 0 indicate significant moderation

$\beta_3(t)$,across age. These results were based on Model 4.5, which is specified above (see Appendix for the corresponding syntax).

To increase interpretability, we plotted the age-varying association between MDD and GAD for male and female individuals on the same figure. Specifically, this model estimates the effect of past-year MDD on past-year GAD separately by sex. Model results can be viewed in Fig. 4.6: the solid green line and associated 95% confidence intervals represent the estimated effect of MDD on GAD for male individuals, and the dashed purple line and associated 95% confidence intervals represent the estimated effect of MDD on GAD for female individuals. As the confidence bands do not include 1.0 across age for either sex, it is clear that this association is significant and positive at all ages for both sexes. In other words, at all ages, individuals of both sexes who meet criteria for MDD are also at increased odds of meeting criteria for GAD across all ages.

We can also use model results presented in Fig. 4.5 to examine differences in the strength of association between MDD and GAD by sex. As originally shown in the interaction plot (Fig. 4.5), significant differences by sex were detected in the covariation of MDD and GAD among adults approximately aged 45–59. As shown in Fig. 4.6, for male adults, the association steadily increases with age among adults aged 18–27, is constant among adults ages 27–39, and then has a fairly sharp increase with age among adults ages 39–57 (peak OR of 15.46 at age 57). The association then weakens across age among male adults ages 57 and older. For female adults however this association is relatively stable across age, increasing slightly across age between ages 23 and 65, with peak levels at age 65 (OR = 8.33). Ages at

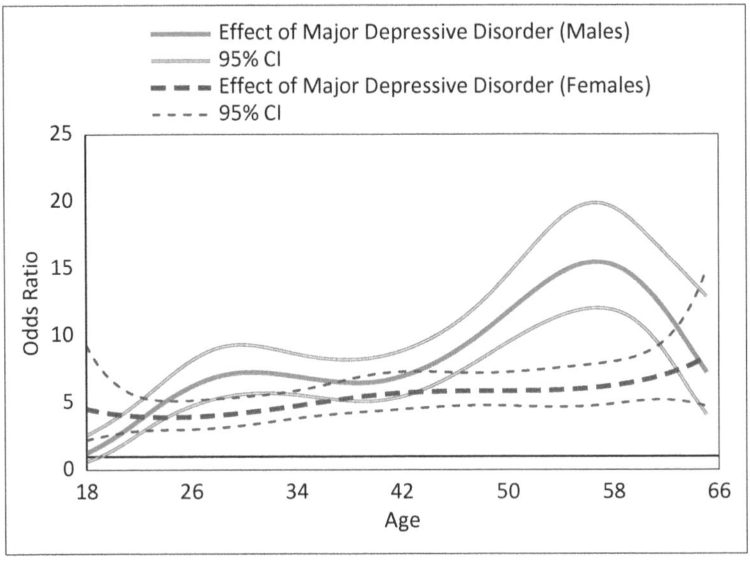

Fig. 4.6 The age-varying association between major depressive disorder and generalized anxiety disorder across age separately for male and female adults as a function of age

which the confidence bands for male and female adults do not overlap indicate ages at which the association is significantly different by sex. However, as discussed in Chaps. 2 and 3, this test tends to be overly conservative. In determining significant moderation by age, results from Model 4.5 (shown in Fig. 4.5) should be used.

4.4 Conclusions

The current study examined the prevalence of past-year GAD and past-year MDD, as well as the association between MDD and GAD, across ages 18–65 and by sex. Findings suggested that while the prevalence of GAD remained somewhat stable across age, MDD decreased somewhat across age. MDD and GAD were highly comorbid across age, and this association was strongest among older adults. Further, while male older adults had a lower prevalence of GAD than female older adults, for male older adults MDD and GAD were more strongly linked. TVEM has an advantage over examining traditionally parsed age groups in epidemiological studies (e.g., 18–30, 30–45, 45–60, 60+), as it revealed changes in prevalence and associations across continuous age. For example, when examining prevalence rates of past-year MDD across all individuals aged 18–65, the prevalence of MDD was highest among individuals approximately age 60 but was at its second-lowest prevalence at age 65. If researchers had collapsed 60- and 65-year-olds into one coarse age group, this drop-off in prevalence would have been missed.

It is important to note that cross-sectional designs have the potential for cohort effects to be confounded with age effects; this prohibits us from making any causal or longitudinal inferences. With a longitudinal dataset, TVEM could however be used to model changes in comorbidity across age within a group of individuals across time. Despite limitations, this study demonstrates the utility of TVEM for assessing changes in associations across age and how individual characteristics moderate these age-varying associations. Chapter 5 showcases another way TVEM can examine changes across time, specifically changes in behavior across historical time.

References

American Psychiatric Association. (2013). *Diagnostic and statistical manual of mental disorders (DSM-5®)*. American Psychiatric Pub.

Amirkhan, J., & Auyeung, B. (2007). Coping with stress across the lifespan: Absolute vs. relative changes in strategy. *Journal of Applied Developmental Psychology, 28*(4), 298–317.

Flannery, K. M., Vannucci, A., & Ohannessian, C. M. (2018). Using time-varying effect modeling to examine age-varying gender differences in coping throughout adolescence and emerging adulthood. *Journal of Adolescent Health, 62*(3), S27–S34.

Grant, B. F., Chu, A., Sigman, R., Amsbary, M., Kali, J., Sugawara, Y., Jiao, R., Ren, W., & Goldstein, R. (2014). *Source and accuracy statement: National Epidemiologic Survey on Alcohol and Related Conditions-III (NESARC-III)* (pp. 1–125). National Institute on Alcohol Abuse and Alcoholism.

Grant, B. F., Goldstein, R. B., Chou, S. P., Saha, T. D., Ruan, W. J., Huang, B., et al. (2011). *The alcohol use disorder and associated disabilities interview schedule-Diagnostic and statistical manual of mental disorders, Fifth edition version (AUDADIS-5)*. National Institute on Alcohol Abuse and Alcoholism.

Grant, B. F., Goldstein, R. B., Smith, S. M., Jung, J., Zhang, H., Chou, S. P., Pickering, R. P., Ruan, W. J., Huang, B., Saha, T. D., Aivadyan, C., Greenstein, E., & Hasin, D. S. (2015). The alcohol use disorder and associated disabilities interview Schedule-5 (AUDADIS-5): Reliability of substance use and psychiatric disorder modules in a general population sample. *Drug and Alcohol Dependence, 148*, 27–33.

Hasin, D. S., Greenstein, E., Aivadyan, C., Stohl, M., Aharonovich, E., Saha, T., Goldstein, R., Nunes, E., Jung, J., Zhang, H., & Grant, B. (2015). The alcohol use disorder and associated disabilities interview Schedule-5 (AUDADIS-5): Procedural validity of substance use disorders modules through clinical re-appraisal in a general population sample. *Drug and Alcohol Dependence, 148*, 40–46.

Linden-Carmichael, A. N., Vasilenko, S. A., Lanza, S. T., & Maggs, J. L. (2017). High-intensity drinking versus heavy episodic drinking: Prevalence rates and relative odds of alcohol use disorder across adulthood. *Alcoholism: Clinical and Experimental Research, 41*(10), 1754–1759.

Moffitt, T. E., Harrington, H., Caspi, A., Kim-Cohen, J., Goldberg, D., Gregory, A. M., Poulton, R. (2007). Depression and generalized anxiety disorder: Cumulative and sequential comorbidity in a birth cohort followed prospectively to age 32 years. *Archives of General Psychiatry, 64*(6), 651–660.

Chapter 5
Time-Varying Effect Modeling to Study Historical Change

5.1 Examining Differences in Associations Across Historical Time Using TVEM

One useful application of time-varying effect modeling (TVEM) is to investigate historical time trends in the mean level or prevalence of an outcome and to examine historical time trends in associations of covariates with an outcome. For example, TVEM could be used to examine perceptions of risk and availability of cannabis in the years leading up to and after cannabis legalization or to examine sex differences in the number of bachelor's degrees awarded in science, technology, engineering, and mathematics across the past few decades. Such examinations require the researcher to have data spanning a historical period and require that the same measurement of the construct was used throughout the time period. If one has data from only a few times in history, TVEM is not needed to examine the time-varying level/prevalence of an outcome or associations. Rather, one could specify a regression model that includes a main effect for time and—if called for—a main effect of a covariate and the interaction between time and the covariate. This parameterization would suffice for showing, for example, linear time trends across three or more points of support (i.e., three or more time points at which the researcher has data).

Possible applications of TVEM for historical time include the analysis of long-running surveys that assess a particular population (e.g., high school seniors) every year for many years, the analysis of health care records that include data from multiple patients or providers across a large time window, and government data presenting historical data on, for example, county-level rates of alcohol tax increases, arrests, motor vehicle accidents, and alcohol-related mortality. One published example used TVEM to examine historical trends from 1976 to 2013 in high school seniors' recent substance use and associations between cannabis use and use of

S. T. Lanza, A. N. Linden-Carmichael, *Time-Varying Effect Modeling for the Behavioral, Social, and Health Sciences*,
https://doi.org/10.1007/978-3-030-70944-0_5

other substances (Lanza, Vasilenko, Dziak, & Butera, 2015). Sex and race (White vs. Black) were then examined as moderators of time-varying associations. This study relied on public use data from the Monitoring the Future (MTF; Johnston, O'Malley, Bachman, Schulenberg, & Miech, 2014; Miech et al., 2020) study, a national, cross-sectional study that was repeated every year beginning in 1976. A variable indicating the year of data collection (e.g., "1976") was appended to each dataset, case identifiers were modified so that each value could uniquely identify both the individual and the year of data collection (i.e., cohort), and common variables assessing substance use were identified across all years and renamed, when necessary, to be consistent across all datasets. The data from each year were then aggregated into a single file using a long format, with one record per individual per year. This unusually large final dataset contained nearly 600,000 records. Findings from this study showed that the prevalence of recent cannabis use peaked in the 1970s then declined through 1990. In recent years however not only is the prevalence of cannabis use rising again, but there is a growing disparity across racial groups such that Black youth are at increasing risk of cannabis use overall, as well as the use of both cannabis and cigarettes.

In this chapter, we present an example similar to the study reported by Lanza et al. (2015). We walk the reader through the specific research questions, describe features of the data, and present equations for the specific models conducted to address each research question (along with syntax in our online Appendix on the companion website, https://prevention.psu.edu/books/tvem/).

5.1.1 Research Questions

In the current study, we use TVEM and MTF data on substance use reported by high school seniors to examine historical trends in the prevalence of recent cigarette use among high school seniors and the associations between cigarette use and (a) sex and (b) perceived level of risk associated with cigarette smoking. We address the following questions:

Research Question 1: What are the historical time trends from 1990 to 2017 in the prevalence of high school seniors who perceive cigarette smoking as high risk and in the prevalence of seniors who report recent cigarette use?

Research Question 2: How do associations between recent cigarette use and (a) sex and (b) perceived risk of smoking change from 1990 to 2017 among high school seniors?

Research Question 3: How does sex moderate, across historical time, the association between perceived risk of smoking and recent cigarette use?

5.2 Method

5.2.1 Sample

The MTF study is an ongoing, annual, cross-sectional survey of high school seniors conducted via in-school surveys. The sample was drawn through a multistage, school-based random sampling strategy. Sampling weights can be used to correct for unequal probability of selection and to ensure representativeness for the 48 continental states. Across years of data collection, the response rate ranged from 77% to 86%.

Data analyzed in this study on recent smoking were from high school seniors (Grade 12) who were surveyed between the years of 1990 and 2017 and were randomly selected to receive Form 3 of the questionnaire, which included a question on perceived risk of cigarette smoking. Data collected from seniors between 1976 and 1989 ($n = 47{,}376$) were excluded because the questionnaire item on perceived risk was not asked until 1990. The resulting total sample size was $n = 68{,}422$; the sample size from each of the 28 years ranged from $n = 2109$ (in 2016) to $n = 2775$ (in 1993). Participants were balanced on sex (weighted 48.6% male).

5.2.2 Measures

Recent cigarette use, the outcome in this study, was assessed with the questionnaire item asking, "How frequently have you smoked cigarettes during the past 30 days?" Response options ranged from 1 (not at all) to 7 (two packs or more per day). Because of the preponderance of nonsmokers (approximately 73%) and extreme skew of the response distribution, recent smoking was coded 0 if participants reported no cigarette smoking during the past 30 days (i.e., response category 1) and 1 if they reported any smoking (i.e., response categories 2 through 7). Perceived risk of smoking was assessed with one item asking, "How much do you think people risk harming themselves (physically or in other ways), if they smoke one or more packs of cigarettes per day?" Response options were 1 for no risk, 2 for slight risk, 3 for moderate risk, and 4 for great risk (individuals who reported 5 for "Can't say/drug unfamiliar" were coded as missing on the indicator for high perceived risk). Because of the high left skew of the response distribution, we created a binary indicator for *high perceived risk* coded as 0 if they reported no, slight, or moderate perceived risk associated with smoking and coded as 1 if they reported great risk. An indicator for sex was coded 1 for male and 0 for female. The distribution of *year*, the "time" variable used in the analysis, was very flat across all years (1990–2017); in other words, the sample size was spread across years fairly evenly. Year was centered at 2000 thus years assessed ranged from −10 (year 1990) to 17 (year 2017) for this analysis so that the span of values in this analysis covered the zero point thus greatly facilitating interpretation (refer to Chap. 2 for a discussion on centering the time axis).

5.2.3 Statistical Analysis

Similar to Chap. 4, estimates for all descriptive statistics and models were weighted using sample weights. A series of weighted logistic time-varying effect models was specified to estimate regression coefficients as a function of historical time. The companion website for this book (https://prevention.psu.edu/books/tvem/) shows the statistical model and syntax used to specify each time-varying effect model used to address the research questions in this study; model numbers used below correspond to those on the website to aid the reader. Also similar to Chap. 4, for research questions that aim to estimate prevalence across levels of covariates, we manually transformed the coefficient functions to reflect prevalence for the purpose of plotting results. These transformations are documented in the Appendix on the companion website (https://prevention.psu.edu/books/tvem/).

Our analytic strategy to address the goals of this study included the estimation of five models. To address Research Question 1 (to examine historical time trends in the prevalence of high school seniors perceiving smoking as high risk and the prevalence of seniors reporting recent cigarette use), Model 5.1 specified an intercept-only TVEM to estimate the prevalence of past 30-day smoking as a nonparametric function of continuous time in years. In addition, Model 5.2 specified an intercept-only TVEM to estimate the prevalence of high perceived risk of smoking as a nonparametric function of continuous time in years. To address Research Question 2 (the association between recent cigarette use, sex, and perceived risk across historical time), Model 5.3 estimated the time-varying association between sex and past 30-day smoking. Similarly, Model 5.4 estimated the time-varying association between perceived smoking risk on recent smoking. Finally, to address Research Question 3 (sex as a moderator of the association between perceived risk and recent cigarette use across historical time), Model 5.5 estimated the odds of past 30-day smoking as a function of sex, high perceived risk of smoking, and their interaction. Despite the fact that the moderator, sex, was not a time-varying covariate (indeed, the model was estimated using repeated cross-sectional data), the moderating effect of this variable was specified to be time-varying thus allowing an examination of the moderating effect of sex on the perceived risk-smoking association as a function of historical time.

As each model incorporated sample weights, B-spline estimation was used. This estimation approach requires the analyst to conduct model selection manually, which we did for each model based on comparing the Akaike information criterion (AIC) and Bayesian information criterion (BIC) across different numbers of knots in the coefficient functions (not shown). Chapter 2 covers estimation, including weighted estimation, as well as selecting the optimal number of knots (corresponding to the optimal complexity of each coefficient function) using the AIC and BIC.

5.3 Results

5.3.1 Research Question 1: What are the Historical Time Trends From 1990 to 2017 in the Prevalence of High School Seniors Who Perceive Cigarette Smoking as High Risk and in the Prevalence of Seniors Who Report Recent Cigarette Use?

The overall weighted estimate of the prevalence of past 30-day cigarette use among MTF high school senior participants sampled from 1990 to 2017 was 24.7% (the rate of missingness on this item was 3.5%). In Fig. 5.1, the solid line represents the estimated prevalence of recent smoking, and the dashed lines show the corresponding 95% confidence band as a function of historical time. Across this time period, the prevalence of recent smoking peaked at approximately 36% in 1997 and then decreased steadily to about 10% in 2017. These results were derived from Model 5.1 (see the online Appendix on the companion website (https://prevention.psu.edu/books/tvem/) for the model specification and corresponding syntax).

Combining participants from all years, the majority of participants reported high perceived risk of cigarette smoking (67.7%; the rate of missingness on this item was 4.0%). Figure 5.2 presents, as a function of historical time, the estimated prevalence of high school seniors reporting high perceived risk of smoking and the corresponding 95% confidence bands. The prevalence of high perceived risk of smoking has

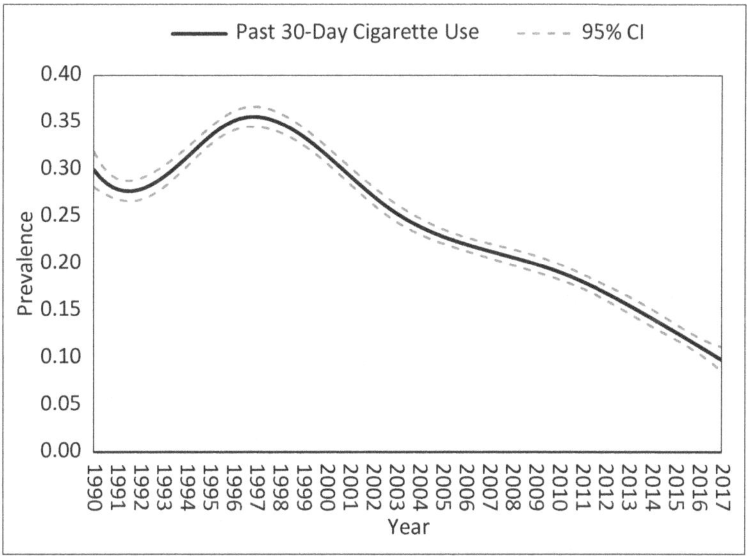

Fig. 5.1 Estimated prevalence (with 95% confidence band) of past 30-day cigarette use among high school students as a function of historical time: 1990–2017

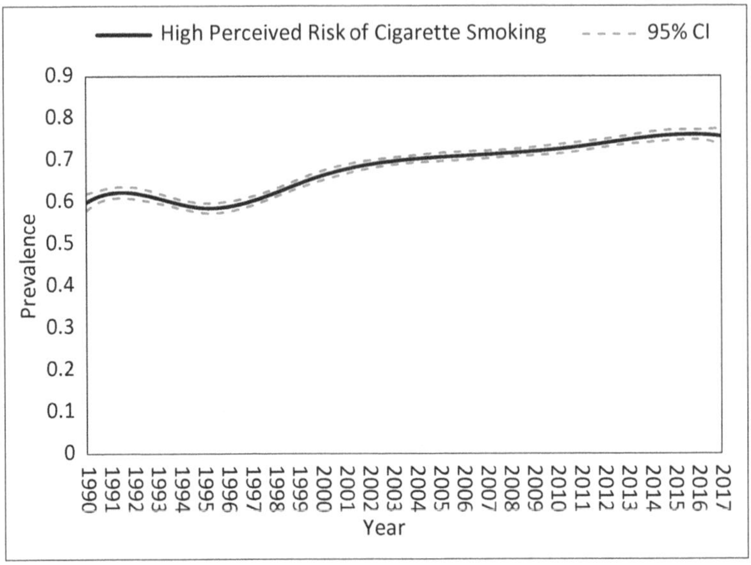

Fig. 5.2 Estimated prevalence (with 95% confidence band) of perceived high risk of cigarette use among high school students as a function of historical time: 1990–2017

increased slowly and steadily over the 28-year period, rising from about 60% in 1990 to 76% in 2017. These results were derived from Model 5.2 (see the online Appendix on the companion website (https://prevention.psu.edu/books/tvem/).

5.3.2 *Research Question 2: How Do Associations Between Recent Cigarette Use and (a) Sex and (b) Perceived Risk Associated With Cigarette Smoking Change From 1990 to 2017 Among High School Seniors?*

Figure 5.3a shows the exponentiated regression coefficient function, or odds ratios (ORs), expressing the association between sex (coded 0 for female and 1 for male) and recent cigarette use as a function of historical time. The upper and lower limits of the 95% confidence intervals are marked with dashed lines. The association is statistically significant ($p < 0.05$) at the times at which the confidence interval does not include the value 1 (marked by the horizontal straight line). This figure shows that the association between sex and recent cigarette use was significant after 1991, with a significant and positive association suggesting that male high school seniors had significantly higher odds of past 30-day cigarette use than female seniors, particularly in more recent years. The year with the strongest association, 2015, has an OR of 1.4, indicating that male seniors had 40% higher odds of recent cigarette use compared to female seniors in that year.

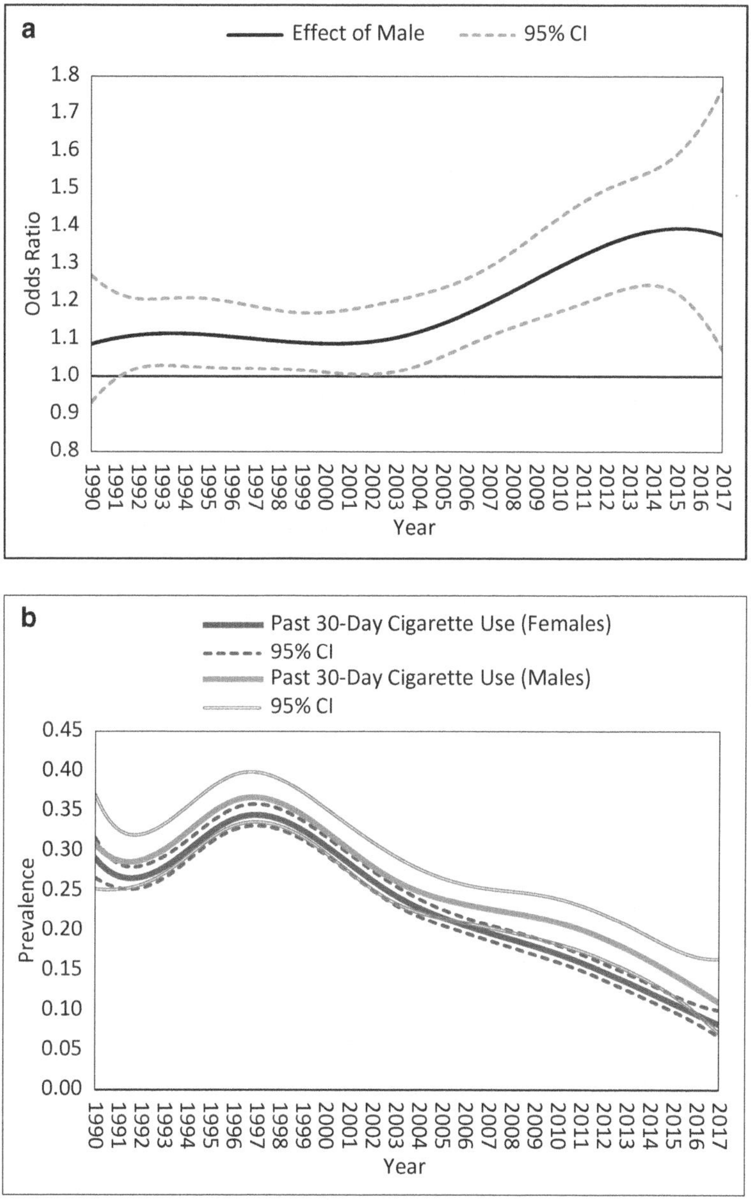

Fig. 5.3 (**a**) Estimated change in odds of past 30-day cigarette smoking (with 95% confidence band) associated with being male. (**b**) Prevalence of past 30-day cigarette smoking (with 95% confidence band) for female and male high school students as a function of historical time: 1990–2017

Shown another way, we further transformed results in Model 5.3 by examining the prevalence of recent cigarette use by sex (Fig. 5.3b; equations shown in the online Appendix on the companion website (https://prevention.psu.edu/books/tvem/)). This type of transformation provides an effective, interpretable way of presenting the results from a time-varying regression coefficient expressing the association between a *categorical* covariate and a *categorical* outcome. The estimated time-varying prevalence of recent cigarette use by sex, along with their corresponding 95% confidence bands, can be viewed in Fig. 5.3b. The prevalence of past 30-day smoking peaked around 1997 for both sexes, with an estimated prevalence of 36.7% among male individuals and 34.5% among female individuals. By 2017, this prevalence dropped substantially to 11.0% among male individuals and 8.2% among female individuals. Time periods when the male and female confidence bands are nonoverlapping do indicate periods where the prevalence is significantly different across groups, but this is a conservative indication of statistical significance (more discussion on this topic is presented in Chap. 3). Instead, statistically significant results from Fig. 5.3a (ORs) should be relied on to determine periods of time during which there was a statistically significant sex difference in the prevalence of cigarette use.

Similar to Fig. 5.3a, which presented the time-varying OR corresponding to sex, Fig. 5.4a presents the time-varying OR representing the association between high perceived risk of smoking and recent cigarette use. Interpreting the OR function, as opposed to the coefficient function prior to exponentiating the values, facilitates the interpretation of this association. These results were derived from Model 5.4 (see the online Appendix on the companion website (https://prevention.psu.edu/books/tvem/)). The association between perceived risk and recent cigarette use was statistically significant and negative across all years examined in this study, with the OR ranging between approximately 0.4 in 2012 and 0.5 in 1990. Overall, this association was quite stable across time. Specifically, the odds of recent cigarette use among individuals who perceive smoking as a high-risk behavior are about half of the odds of cigarette use among individuals who do not perceive smoking to have high health risks.

Figure 5.4b shows results from Model 5.4 that were further transformed, providing the estimated prevalence of recent cigarette use (and corresponding 95% confidence bands) for high school seniors with higher and lower perceived smoking risk. We first comment on the direction of the effect: at all years included in this investigation, high school seniors who perceive smoking as having high risk have a substantially lower prevalence of recent cigarette use. Next, we note that the shapes of the time trends in past 30-day smoking are similar, rising during the early- to mid-1990s and then declining throughout the most recent 15 years. We then interpret more specific features of the estimated time trends. Specifically, among students who perceive smoking as a high-risk behavior, the prevalence of recent cigarette use peaked at 0.27 around 1997 and has fallen to less than 0.08 in 2017

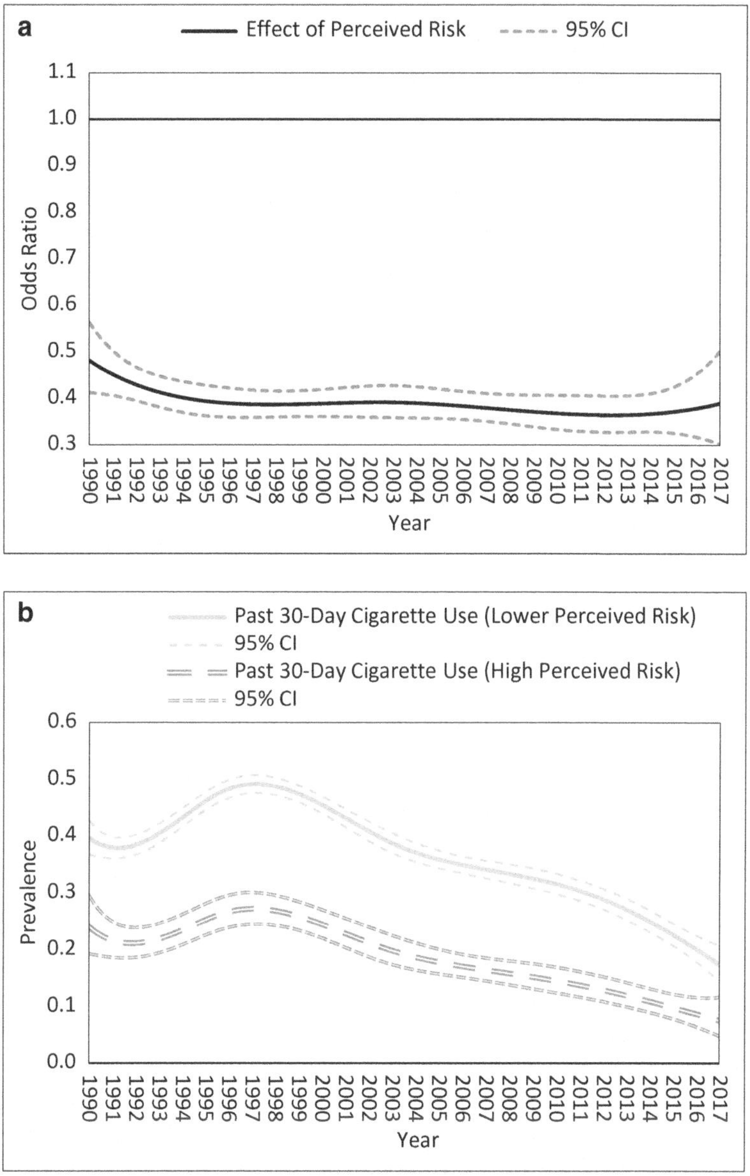

Fig. 5.4 (**a**) Estimated change in odds of past 30-day cigarette smoking (with 95% confidence band) associated with high perceived risk of cigarette use. (**b**) Prevalence of past 30-day cigarette smoking (with 95% confidence band) for high school students with high and lower perceived risk of smoking as a function of historical time: 1990–2017

(dashed red line in Fig. 5.4b). In contrast, among students who do not perceive smoking as high risk, the prevalence of recent cigarette use peaked at 0.49 around 1997 and fell to 0.17 in 2017 (solid blue line in Fig. 5.4b).

5.3.3 Research Question 3: How Does Sex Moderate, Across Historical Time, the Association Between Perceived Risk of Cigarette Smoking and Recent Cigarette Use?

Finally, Model 5.5 was used to test for a time-varying moderation effect of sex on the association between perceived risk of smoking and recent cigarette use. This final model, also shown in the online Appendix on the companion website (https://prevention.psu.edu/books/tvem/), was specified as

$$ln\left(\frac{P(CIG)}{1+P(CIG)}\right)=\beta_0(t)+\beta_1(t)RISK_i+\beta_2(t)SEX_i+\beta_3(t)RISK\_SEX_i.$$

The coefficient functions $\beta_1(t)$ and $\beta_2(t)$ express the time-varying main effects of perceived smoking risk and sex, respectively. Given the dummy coding of $RISK_i$ and SEX_i, $\beta_1(t)$ represents the time-varying effect of perceived risk for female individuals (where $SEX_i = 0$), and $\beta_2(t)$ represents the time-varying effect of being male among those with lower perceived risk of smoking (where $RISK_i = 0$). Figure 5.5a presents the time-varying effect of the perceived risk-by-sex interaction term, $\beta_3(t)$. Importantly, this coefficient function allows for nuanced hypothesis testing of sex as a moderator of the association between perceived risk and recent smoking. Times at which the coefficient's confidence band does not include the value 0 indicate that sex is a significant moderator of the association. Thus, Fig. 5.5 indicates that significant sex differences were detected between 2004 and 2009.

To further parse out this interaction, Fig. 5.5b shows information from the Model 5.5 estimates, transformed to facilitate interpretation of the interaction term. The time-varying prevalence of recent cigarette use was calculated for each of four groups: (1) female, perceive smoking as high risk; (2) female, perceive smoking as lower risk; (3) male, perceive smoking as high risk; and (4) male, perceive smoking as lower risk. This figure conveys the overwhelmingly large differences across levels of perceived smoking risk compared to the differences associated with being male or female. It also adds context to the finding that the association between perceived smoking risk and recent cigarette use was not different by sex during many of the years studied, but that in fairly recent years the gap between cigarette use prevalences for those with high versus lower perceived smoking risk has decreased among high school students.

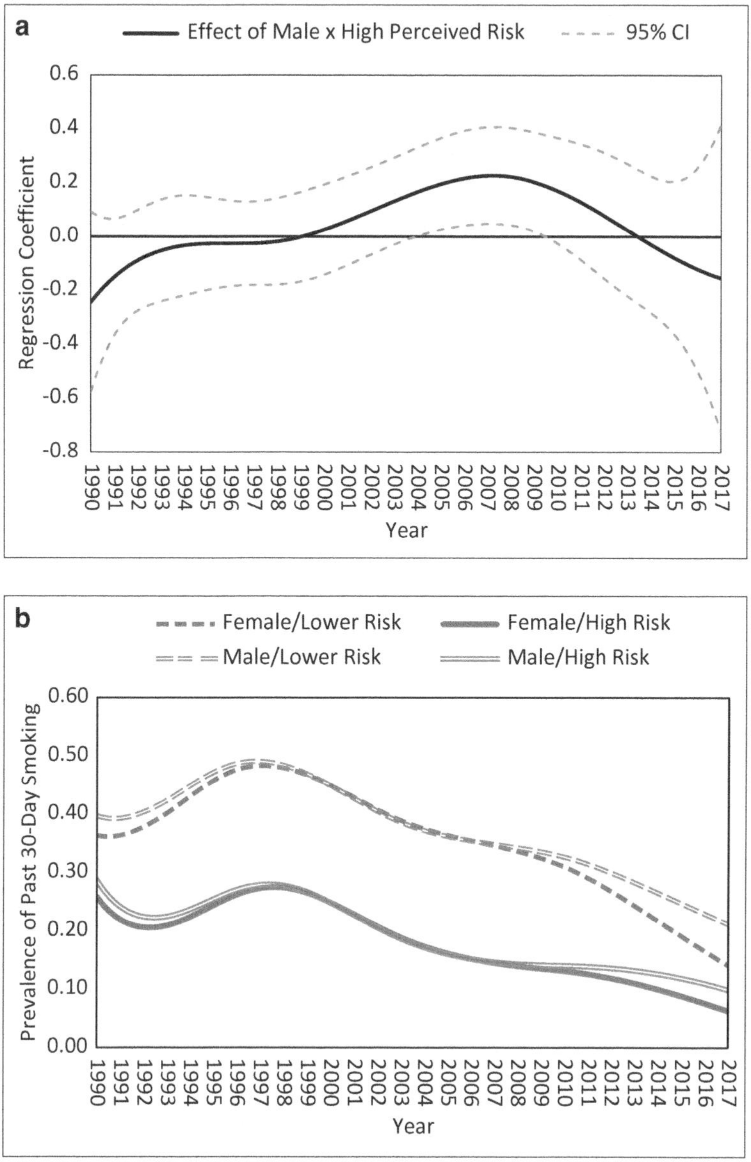

Fig. 5.5 (**a**) Age-varying coefficient for the interaction between male and high perceived risk predicting past 30-day cigarette use. Years at which the confidence interval does not include 0 indicate significant moderation. (**b**) Age-varying prevalences of past 30-day cigarette use among high school students given sex and perceived smoking risk as a function of historical time: 1990–2017

5.4 Conclusions

This study applied TVEM to study historical trends in recent cigarette use and its perceived risk, as well as historical trends in links of recent cigarette use with sex and perceived risk of smoking. It is conceivable that one could map data from other sources onto historical data such as this to answer additional questions. For example, if a federal policy change or a public health awareness campaign was initiated at a particular time point covered in the study, one could specify a discrete curve shift in the time trend in the prevalence of smoking as well as its association with covariates. This can be done by adding a time-varying covariate that reflects whether that particular year was prior to or after the event (i.e., coded 0 for all years prior to the event, and 1 for all years after). Then, this *time-varying covariate* could be added to the model and specified to have a *time-invariant effect*. A significant effect would reflect a curve shift corresponding to that year, which may be in part due to the occurrence of the event.

The study has limitations, including the fact that any trends in links between the covariates and recent smoking must be interpreted as within-time associations; the repeated cross-sectional study design does not permit causality or directionality to be inferred. Further, because of the design, time lags cannot be specified to examine whether, historically, shifts in perceived risk of smoking occur nationally prior to behavior changes. However, despite these limitations, this study demonstrates how historical data that include multiple measures used consistently across a period of time can be modeled with TVEM to better describe nuanced time trends, as well as historical shifts in associations between variables.

We hope the current study enables readers to conceive of new historical-change questions of scientific interest that can be addressed using TVEM. In Chap. 6, we turn to another application of TVEM, demonstrating its use to examine change across real-time using intensive longitudinal data.

References

Johnston, L. D., O'Malley, P. M., Bachman, J. G., Schulenberg, J. E., & Miech, R. A. (2014). *Monitoring the Future: National survey results on drug use, 1975–2013: Volume I, secondary school students*. Institute for Social Research, University of Michigan.

Lanza, S. T., Vasilenko, S. A., Dziak, J. J., & Butera, N. M. (2015). Trends among US high school seniors in recent marijuana use and associations with other substances: 1976–2013. *Journal of Adolescent Health, 57*(2), 198–204.

Miech, R., Johnston, L., O'Malley, P., Bachman, J., Schulenberg, J., & Patrick, M. (2020). *Monitoring the Future national survey results on drug use, 1975–2019: Volume I, secondary school students*. Institute for Social Research, University of Michigan.

Chapter 6
Time-Varying Effect Modeling for Intensive Longitudinal Data

6.1 TVEM for Intensive Longitudinal Data

Throughout this book, we have provided examples of how time-varying effect modeling (TVEM) can be applied to cross-sectional, longitudinal, and historical data, but TVEM was originally developed for analyzing intensive longitudinal data (ILD). ILD are data with many measurements over time. New technologies like smartphones and fitness trackers are generating massive amounts of passively collected (i.e., collected in the background without requiring individuals' active input) ILD that are relevant to social, health, and behavioral research. These technologies also provide new opportunities to actively collect survey data with frequent assessments in the context of real-life, including daily diary data and ecological momentary assessments (EMA). ILD have a unique capacity to capture both central tendency and variability within an individual. For example, EMA collected on a person's mood at the moment can provide an indication both of their overall or typical mood and the size and suddenness of their mood fluctuations. Importantly, by also capturing key time-varying contextual factors in real-time, ILD provide immense opportunity to study risk factors and mechanisms that may operate both across and within individuals. As data collection technology such as smartphones and actigraph devices create richer and denser datasets, TVEM can enable researchers to answer new and more nuanced questions than was possible just a few years ago. This applies to many fields of study where ILD are being collected, including in behavioral science (e.g., smoking, eating behavior, substance use), social science (e.g., cognitive functioning, positive and negative affect), and other fields of health research (e.g., the course of HIV and other diseases and adherence to medication).

When analyzing ILD, analysts usually turn to multilevel modeling (MLM, also referred to as mixed effects modeling, random effects modeling, and hierarchical linear modeling). MLM is an extremely useful approach that adjusts standard errors to account for the clustering of repeated observations within individuals. MLM also

S. T. Lanza, A. N. Linden-Carmichael, *Time-Varying Effect Modeling for the Behavioral, Social, and Health Sciences*,
https://doi.org/10.1007/978-3-030-70944-0_6

partitions the variance in an outcome into between-person variance (the degree to which people differ from each other on average) and within-person variance (the degree to which people differ from themselves across repeated assessments). MLM allows researchers to model the effects of covariates at both the between-person and within-person levels. Although MLM is a powerful and flexible approach that allows users to specify a wide range of models and to address diverse research questions using ILD, multilevel models can be specified in a way that detects change over time in an outcome (typically as a strict parametric function of time, such as linear) and accommodates time-varying covariates, but that typically assumes any associations between covariates and the outcome are constant across time. For example, in a smoking cessation trial in which individuals' nicotine craving and negative affect were assessed repeatedly after a quit attempt, in MLM the association between negative affect and nicotine craving typically would be assumed to be constant across the entire post-quit time interval. TVEM allows analysts to explore the possibility that associations do, in fact, change as flexible functions of time and that the shape of change over time may be highly complex. For example, attempts to quit smoking are influenced by a broad range of factors, including mood, belief in one's ability to quit, and stress level. Further, these time-varying associations may differ as a function of baseline characteristics such as intervention condition. As briefly discussed in Chap. 3, TVEM has been used to examine dynamic outcomes such as craving, as well as dynamic associations between craving and time-varying covariates such as negative affect, as a function of both time since smoking quit attempt and intervention condition (Lanza, Vasilenko, Liu, Li, & Piper, 2014; Vasilenko et al., 2014). These analyses added to the understanding of smoking cessation attempts beyond what had been learned using MLM to analyze the same data, including providing insight into when during a quit attempt an individual might require additional support in order to succeed.

There are several considerations when using TVEM to analyze ILD. First, ILD inherently has a multilevel structure, such that many occasions are nested within individuals. Second, while there is no hard and fast rule about the number of assessments needed from each individual, a sufficient number of data points are needed to capture change over time in the process being studied. In other words, the more dynamic and complex the relationship being modeled, the more valuable it is to have longitudinal data collected more intensively (and, thus, with better coverage of the time axis). Finally, as always in TVEM, a meaningful interpretation for 0 on the time variable is required. This is important when modeling ILD, as in some instances TVEM may not be appropriate. For example, many EMA studies are designed to purposefully collect data at random moments of time during an individual's normal life; in this case, the only meaningful zero point might be the start of the study. However, if systematic change across time in study is not of interest, TVEM is likely not the right technique. Even in studies that are designed to sample participants at randomly selected times, it may be the case that the data can be used to address research questions that conceive of time differently, such as time relative to an observed event. In the empirical example we present below, we considered the "zero point" of time to be the first day on which an interparental conflict event was reported during a predetermined assessment period (in this case, a 15-day period during the daily diary study). For each individual, then, the variable indicating day was recoded (e.g., Day = −1 corresponds to the day prior to the conflict event; Day = 0 reflects the day of the event; Day = 1 corresponds to the day after the event, and so on). It is important to note that whatever the data type, the data must be organized so that 0 on the time variable holds the same meaning for each subject.

6.2 Current Study

In this empirical demonstration of TVEM to model ILD, we analyzed data from a 21-day daily diary study assessing parents' and their adolescents' behaviors and feelings. Traditional MLM could be used to compare days with and without parent-child conflict and examine day-level (e.g., adolescent's current mood) and person-level (e.g., parent-adolescent closeness) covariates associated with the odds of a parent-child conflict event occurring on a given day. Some of the most interesting questions that can be addressed in MLM involve cross-level interactions; that is, interactions between a day-level covariate and a person-level covariate. An example research question involving a cross-level interaction is, "*Does the within-person association between adolescents' current-day mood and the odds of parent-child conflict on that day differ for families with different levels of parent-child closeness?*" TVEM can be used to address somewhat different, complementary questions by incorporating time into the model. Rather than comparing types of days (e.g., days with higher negative affect compared to days with lower negative affect), TVEM can be used to model variables such as mood and behavior—as well as their associations—as a function of time relative to the occurrence of an event. Two such research questions are, "*How do adolescents' moods change across time in the days preceding and following a parent-child conflict event?*" and "*How does mood as a function of time relative to a conflict event differ based on parent-child closeness?*"

As noted above, in the example in this chapter, time is represented by days relative to the first reported interparental conflict event during the specified assessment window. We examined the associations of day-level (parent-child conflict) and person-level (family income, interparental love) covariates with the outcome, interparental conflict, across the study period. Specifically, we had the following research questions:

Research Question 1: How does the mean level of interparental conflict fluctuate across days relative to a reported interparental conflict event (a) without controlling for and (b) while controlling for interparental conflict events on other days?

Research Question 2: How do associations between level of interparental conflict and (a) baseline family income, (b) baseline interparental love, and (c) daily level of parent-child conflict vary across days relative to a reported interparental conflict event after controlling for interparental conflict events on other days?

Research Question 3: Do family income and interparental love moderate the association between daily level of parent-child conflict and daily level of interparental conflict across days relative to a reported interparental conflict event after controlling for other interparental conflict events on other days?

6.3 Method

Data for the current analyses were drawn from the full sample of the Family Life Optimizing Well-being (FLOW) study, a daily diary study wherein parents and their adolescents completed 21 daily reports about family functioning, their feelings, and well-being (Fosco & Lydon-Staley, 2019). The present analyses use only the parent/caregiver reports.

6.3.1 Participants and Procedure

Participants in FLOW included 150 families with two caregivers of 9th- and 10th-grade adolescents recruited through high schools in Pennsylvania. Participating caregivers were between ages 30 and 61 years ($M = 43.35$, $SD = 6.89$) and identified as their adolescent's mother (n = 139), father (n = 7), stepmother (n = 2), aunt (n = 1), or foster mother (n = 1); and as Caucasian (n = 138), African American/Black (n = 6), Native American/American Indian (n = 3), Asian American (n = 5), Latinx (n = 2), and Other (n = 1). Caregivers' education spanned graduate or professional training (n = 35), college degree (n = 42), associate's degree or more than 1 year of college (n = 46), and high school degree or less (n = 26). Median family income was $70,000–$79,999.

Participants were recruited through email sent to parents from school principals and through family referrals. After providing informed consent, eligible caregivers completed a baseline survey that included baseline trait variables and demographic information, and then the daily diary protocol was initiated. For 21 days, links to daily surveys were emailed to caregivers at 7:00 each evening, accompanied by a reminder text message or phone call. Participants were instructed to complete the daily survey before going to bed, although the links remained open until 9:00 the next morning. Daily surveys took approximately 5 min to complete; parents provided an average of 20.3 (96.5%) out of the possible 21 daily reports (range 10–21 days). For additional details on the study protocol, see Fosco and Lydon-Staley (2019).

To be included in the present analysis, families must have reported a conflict event between Day 4 and Day 18 of the study (see Statistical Analysis section below for rationale). From the larger dataset, 97 families met this criterion and thus were examined here. From these 97 families, we analyzed data from 1504 person-days.

6.3.2 Measures

6.3.2.1 Baseline Measures

Interparental love was assessed using five items from the Love subscale from the Love and Relationships scale, with higher scores representing greater levels of interparental love (Braiker & Kelley, 1979). Mean level interparental love was 4.34 (*SD* = 0.92; range 1.40–5.0). *Family income* was assessed at baseline using 12 income brackets ranging from "less than $10,000 annually" to "$125,000 or more." Income was treated as a continuous covariate.

6.3.2.2 Daily Measures

Reported interparental conflict events. Each evening, parents reported whether they experienced a conflict event with their partner by answering the question, "I had a disagreement or argument with my partner ***today,***" with response options of *yes* or *no*. This binary variable was used to center time on the x-axis to reflect days relative to the first reported interparental conflict event in the study, as described in the Statistical Analysis section below. Hereafter, we refer to the first event simply as the "conflict event." A time-varying indicator of interparental conflict events reported on any of the other study days was coded as 1 for an event and 0 otherwise; this was included as a control variable in certain analyses (see Statistical Analysis below).

Daily level of interparental conflict. As part of each evening's questionnaire, parents rated that day's level of conflict between caregivers from 0 (*not at all*) to 10 (*a lot*) in 0.1 increments. Parents responded to two items, "*My partner and I were* ***angry*** *or* ***mad at each other*** *today,*" and "*My partner and I* ***disagreed with each other*** *today.*" Daily interparental conflict scores, calculated as the average of the two items, ranged from 0–10.

Daily level of parent-child conflict. Parents' perception of conflict with their adolescent child was assessed each evening using two items. Parents indicated, using a 0–10 slider, the extent to which they agreed with the statements, "*I was* ***angry*** *or* ***mad*** *at my child,*" and "*There was* ***tension*** *between my child and I [sic] today.*" Daily parent-child conflict scores, calculated as the average of the two items, ranged from 0–10.

6.3.3 Statistical Analysis

The present analysis used all available data from the 21 daily assessments. However, we coded the time axis such that zero corresponded to the first conflict event reported during Days 4–18 of the study. This was done to ensure that there would be at least 3 days of data preceding the conflict event (i.e., Days 1–3 if the first conflict event during Days 4–18 occurred on Day 4) and at least 3 days after the conflict event (i.e., Days 19–21 if the first conflict event during Days 4–18 occurred on Day 18). Since these events occurred at different times for different individuals, time was centered within individuals such that 0 represents the day of the first reported conflict event (during Days 4–18) for each participant. Thus, the time metric (days) could have values ranging from −17 (corresponding to data from Day 1, if the first conflict event was reported on Day 18) to +17 (corresponding to data from Day 21, if the first conflict event was reported on Day 4). After re-centering time within each participant, we examined the coverage of data across the x-axis (days) and opted to limit our analysis to all available data coded between −7 and + 12 days, reflecting the entire week prior to first reported conflict event and 12 days after the conflict event. In order to control for the fact that additional conflict events may have occurred across the study, a time-varying indicator was coded to reflect whether a conflict occurred on days other than the conflict event used to anchor time; this time-varying indicator, coded each day as 1 for a reported conflict event and 0 otherwise, was included in some models as a control variable to adjust for additional conflict events.

Our analytic strategy included estimating seven time-varying effect models. The companion website for this book (https://prevention.psu.edu/books/tvem/) shows the statistical model and syntax used to specify each time-varying effect model used to address the research questions in this study; model numbers used below correspond to those on the website to aid the reader. To address Research Question 1 (to estimate the mean level of interparental conflict across days relative to the conflict event), we estimated an intercept-only model for the mean level of interparental conflict without including the indicator of other conflict events (Model 6.1) and with including the indicator of other conflict events (Model 6.2) as a function of days relative to the event. To address Research Question 2 (the association of level of interparental conflict with day- and person-level covariates), Model 6.3 estimated the time-varying association between a time-invariant covariate, family income, and daily level of interparental conflict across days relative to the event. Similarly, Model 6.4 estimated the time-varying association between interparental love, also a time-invariant covariate, and level of daily interparental conflict. Model 6.5 was specified to model level of interparental conflict as a function of daily level of parent-child conflict; parent-child conflict was a time-varying covariate with an association that was allowed to vary across days relative to first conflict event. Finally, to address Research Question 3 (moderators of the association between parent-child conflict and interparental conflict across days), Models 6.6 and 6.7 estimated family income and interparental love, respectively, as moderators of the time-varying association between level of parent-child conflict and level of interparental conflict across days relative to the event. Both moderation effects were specified as time-varying, allowing us to examine changes in the extent to which moderation was detected over time. To interpret the significant moderation effect of interparental love, simple slopes for the time-varying association between level of parent-child conflict and level of interparental conflict were calculated and plotted for values at 1 *SD* above and below the sample mean of interparental love. With the exception of Model 6.1, the time-varying indicator of other conflict events was included as a covariate in all analyses. A normal distribution was specified for the outcome, and P-spline estimation was used in all analyses.

6.4 Results

6.4.1 Research Question 1: How Does the Mean Level of Interparental Conflict Fluctuate Across Days Relative to a Reported Interparental Conflict Event (a) Without Controlling for and (b) While Controlling for Interparental Conflict Events on Other Days?

An intercept-only TVEM was specified to examine how mean level of daily interparental conflict changes systematically across days leading up to and following the first reported conflict event. Day 0 reflects the day of the event, with negative values indicating the number of days prior to the event and positive values indicating days since the event. As shown in Fig. 6.1, mean level of interparental conflict (e.g., anger toward partner, disagreements with partner) remained fairly low across approximately 4 days (from 7 to 3 days prior to the conflict event), then began to increase markedly in the 3 days immediately before the event. Mean level of conflict then recovered to pre-event levels within about 4 days following the conflict event.

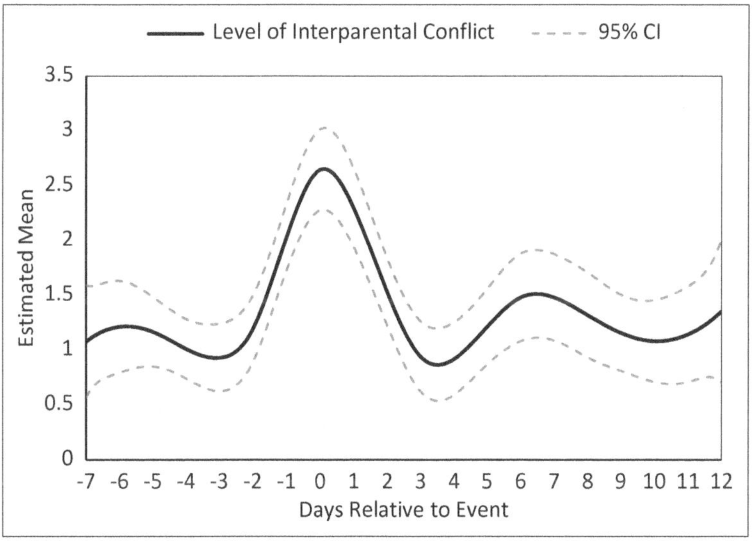

Fig. 6.1 Estimated mean level of interparental conflict across days relative to a reported interparental conflict event (Day 0), without controlling for conflict experienced on other days

Figure 6.2 also estimates the mean level of interparental conflict across days but includes an indicator of conflict experienced on other days. The overall pattern is fairly similar but with tightened confidence intervals, particularly on the earlier and later days of assessment. The equation for Model 6.2 (corresponding to Fig. 6.2) for interparental conflict on Day *d* for individual *i*, controlling for other conflict events, can be expressed as

$$PARENTCONFLICT_{di} = \beta_0(t) + \beta_1(t)OTHERCON_{di} + \varepsilon_{di},$$

where $\beta_0(t)$ represents the time-varying mean level of interparental conflict when no other conflict event is reported, $\beta_1(t)$ represents the time-varying effect of the control variable, and ε_{di} represents the residual for individual *i* on Day *d*.

Figure 6.2 shows a coefficient function that is very similar to Fig. 6.1 in shape, although the interpretation of this intercept function now is the time-varying mean interparental conflict on days with no conflict event, relative to the timing of the key event. Not surprisingly, mean level of conflict is somewhat lower on no conflict days (Fig. 6.2) compared to all days (Fig. 6.1). For completeness, Fig. 6.3 shows the coefficient function for the control variable. In practice, control variables—even those that are time-varying, as in our example—often are specified as having time-invariant effects, and thus a figure would not be produced. This coefficient function shows that the effect of the control variable is statistically significant and strong, such that interparental conflict is expected to be about 4 units higher on days with an additional conflict event than on days without one, and this association is relatively constant across days.

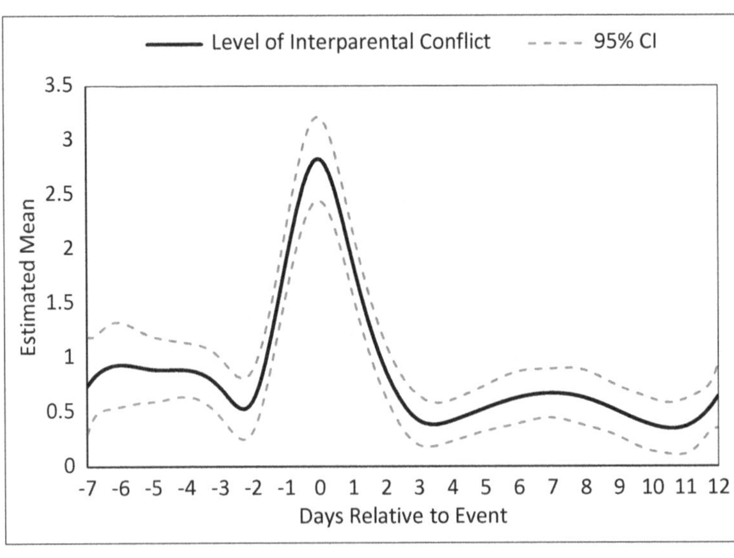

Fig. 6.2 Estimated mean level of interparental conflict across days relative to a reported interparental conflict event (Day 0), holding conflict experienced on other days at 0

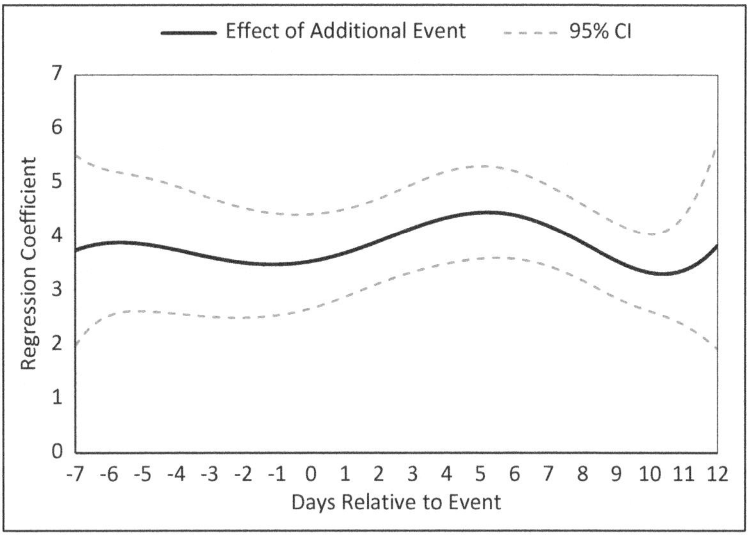

Fig. 6.3 Coefficient function for the time-varying covariate indicating an additional conflict event (i.e., coefficient function for the control variable). Coefficients of 0 indicate no association between additional event and level of interparental conflict

6.4.2 Research Question 2: How Do Associations Between Level of Interparental Conflict and (a) Baseline Family Income, (b) Baseline Interparental Love, and (c) Daily Level of Parent-Child Conflict Vary Across Days Relative to a Reported Interparental Conflict Event After Controlling for Interparental Conflict Events on Other Days?

To address this research question, TVEM was used with three models for level of interparental conflict as the outcome, with family income (Model 6.3), interparental love (Model 6.4), and daily level of parent-child conflict (Model 6.5) examined separately as covariates. All models controlled for the occurrence of other conflict events. As an example, the association between family income and level of interparental conflict across days while controlling for other conflict events was expressed as

$$PARENTCONFLICT_{di} = \beta_0(t) + \beta_1(t)INCOME_i + \beta_2(t)OTHERCON_{di} + \varepsilon_{di}.$$

As demonstrated by confidence intervals that overlap with an estimated association of 0 across most time points in Fig. 6.4, family income generally was not significantly associated with interparental conflict, except on the day of the first conflict event (i.e., Day 0 on the *x*-axis). On the day of the event, higher family income was significantly associated with higher levels of interparental conflict ($B = 0.22$, 95%

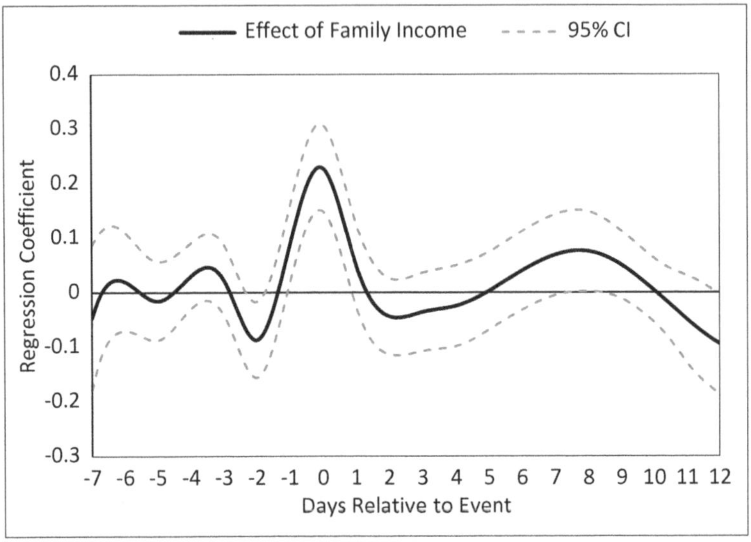

Fig. 6.4 Time-varying association between baseline family income and level of interparental conflict across days relative to a conflict event (Day 0), controlling for conflict experienced on other days (with 95% confidence band)

CI = 0.14–0.30). Additionally, although the effect size was very small, higher income was significantly associated with lower mean levels of interparental conflict 2 days preceding the first conflict event ($B = -0.09$, 95% CI = −0.16–−0.02).

Figure 6.5 shows the association between level of interparental love and level of interparental conflict across days relative to the conflict event. Beginning around 5 days prior to the conflict event through the first 10 days following the event, a higher level of interparental love was associated with a lower level of interparental conflict. This effect was quite constant across time, although confidence intervals on days before 5 days prior to the event and more than 10 days after the event were wider, reducing confidence in findings during these time windows.

Figure 6.6 shows the time-varying association between daily (parent-reported) parent-child conflict and level of interparental conflict across days relative to the conflict event. Across all days, higher levels of parent-child conflict were significantly associated with higher levels of interparental conflict; the size of this effect strengthened over the 5 days preceding the first conflict event and continued to increase through 2 days after the event. The association remained fairly constant across the 12 days after the event, with the strongest association at Day 12 ($B = 0.33$, 95% CI = 0.06–0.59).

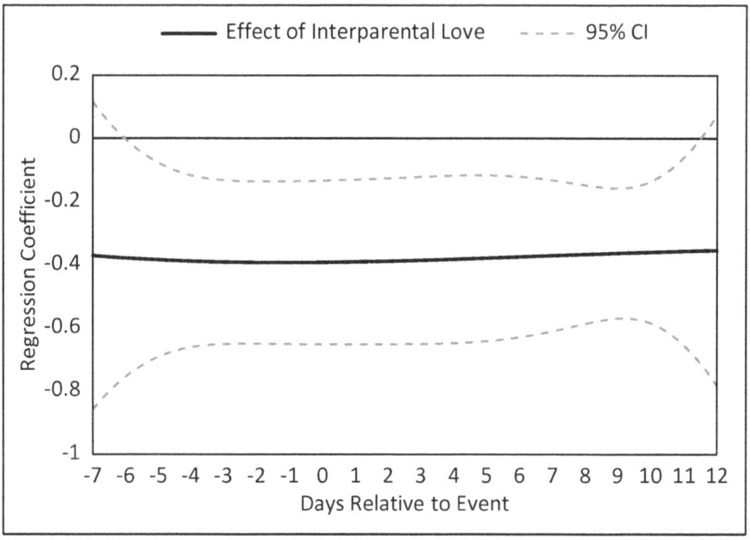

Fig. 6.5 Time-varying association between baseline interparental love and level of interparental conflict across days relative to a conflict event (Day 0), controlling for conflict experienced on other days (with 95% confidence band)

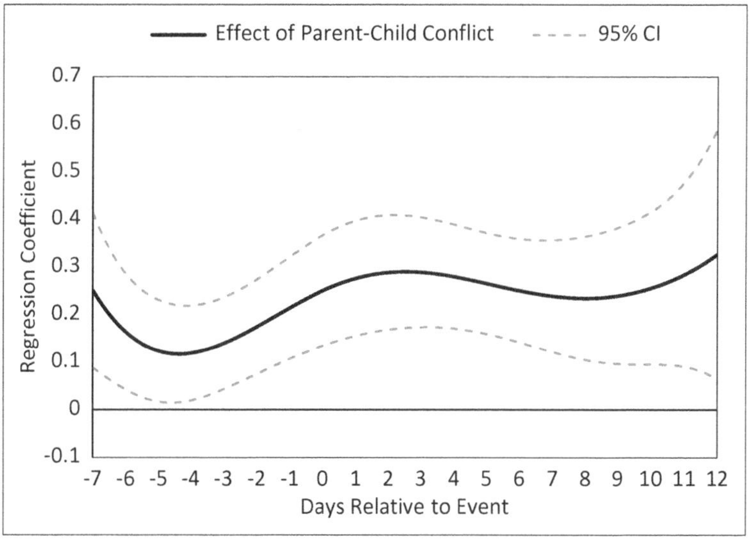

Fig. 6.6 Time-varying association between daily parent-child conflict and level of interparental conflict across days relative to a conflict event (Day 0), controlling for conflict experienced on other days (with 95% confidence band)

6.4.3 Research Question 3: Do Family Income and Interparental Love Moderate the Association Between Daily Level of Parent-Child Conflict and Daily Level of Interparental Conflict Across Days Relative to a Reported Interparental Conflict Event After Controlling for Other Interparental Conflict Events on Other Days?

Our final models examined (a) the effect of the interaction between family income and daily level of parent-child conflict on level of interparental conflict and (b) the effect of the interaction between interparental love and daily level of parent-child conflict on level of interparental conflict, both as time-varying effects relative to day of conflict event. To test the interaction between family income and daily level of parent-child conflict, for example, the model includes coefficients for the intercept, the level of family income (*INCOME*), the level of parent-child conflict (*PC_CONFLICT*), and the interaction between income and parent-child conflict (*INCOME*PC_CONFLICT*), while controlling for other conflict events, in predicting interparental conflict, as follows:

$$PARENTCONFLICT_{di} = \beta_0(t) + \beta_1(t)INCOME_i + \beta_2(t)PC\_CONFLICT_{di} + \beta_3(t)INCOME_i * PC\_CONFLICT_{di} + \beta_4(t)OTHERCON_{di} + \varepsilon_{di}$$

Note that moderators can be measured more than once to assess a time-varying moderator. Figure 6.7 shows the time-varying effect of the interaction between income and level of parent-child conflict when predicting level of interparental conflict across days, controlling for conflict experienced on other days. As shown by confidence intervals that overlap with 0 across all days, the association between level of parent-child conflict and level of interparental conflict is not moderated by level of family income.

Finally, we examined baseline interparental love as a moderator of the association between level of parent-child conflict and level of interparental conflict across days. The interaction effect is presented in Fig. 6.8a; as shown here, the interaction is significant from 4 days leading up to the first conflict event until the day of the event. Examining this more closely, in Fig. 6.8b we see that during this period, parents with higher (1 *SD* above the mean) levels of interparental love (double purple line) had a weaker association between parent-child conflict and interparental conflict than parents with lower (1 *SD* below the mean) levels of interparental love (dashed red line). When focusing only on parents with lower levels of interparental love, the slope is much steeper moving from 4 days before to the day of the event. For those reporting higher levels of interparental love, although interparental conflict increases days leading up to the conflict event, this association shows less of a "spike" on interparental conflict relative to parents with lower levels of interparental

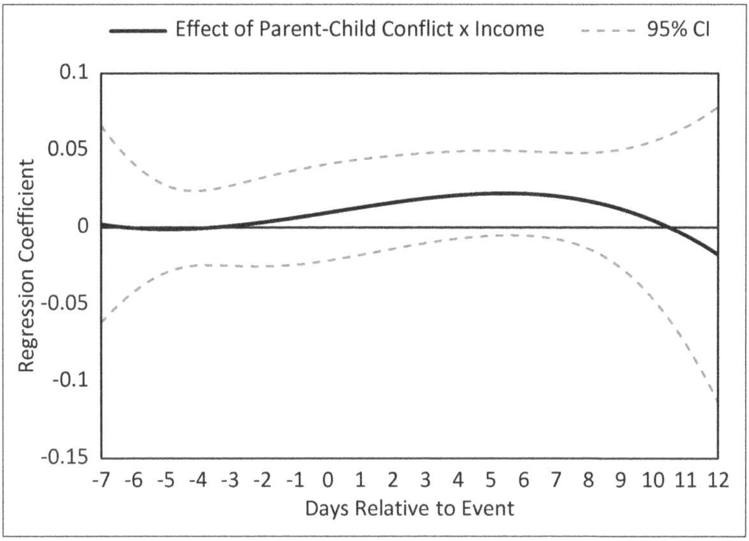

Fig. 6.7 Effect of the interaction between parent-child conflict and family income on interparental conflict across days relative to a conflict event (Day 0), controlling for conflict experienced on other days (with 95% confidence band)

love. Days on which significant differences were observed between parents with higher versus lower levels of interparental love are denoted with a brace in Fig. 6.8b.

6.5 Conclusions

The current study among parents with adolescent children examined the mean level of interparental conflict in the days leading up to and following the first interparental conflict event reported during Days 4–18 of a 21-day assessment period. We also examined the associations between daily level of parent-child conflict, as well as baseline family income and level of interparental love, with level of interparental conflict across days relative to the first conflict event. Findings revealed that levels of interparental conflict increased across approximately 3 days preceding a conflict event, then recovered to preevent levels within approximately 4 days following the event. Family income had a minimal association with day-level interparental conflict, with higher earning families reporting slightly higher levels of conflict on the day of the conflict event. Parents with higher levels of interparental love generally reported lower levels of conflict across days. Daily level of parent-child conflict was found to have a significant and increasing positive association with daily level of interparental conflict across days leading up to the conflict event and several days after the conflict event, but interparental love was found to be a protective factor on

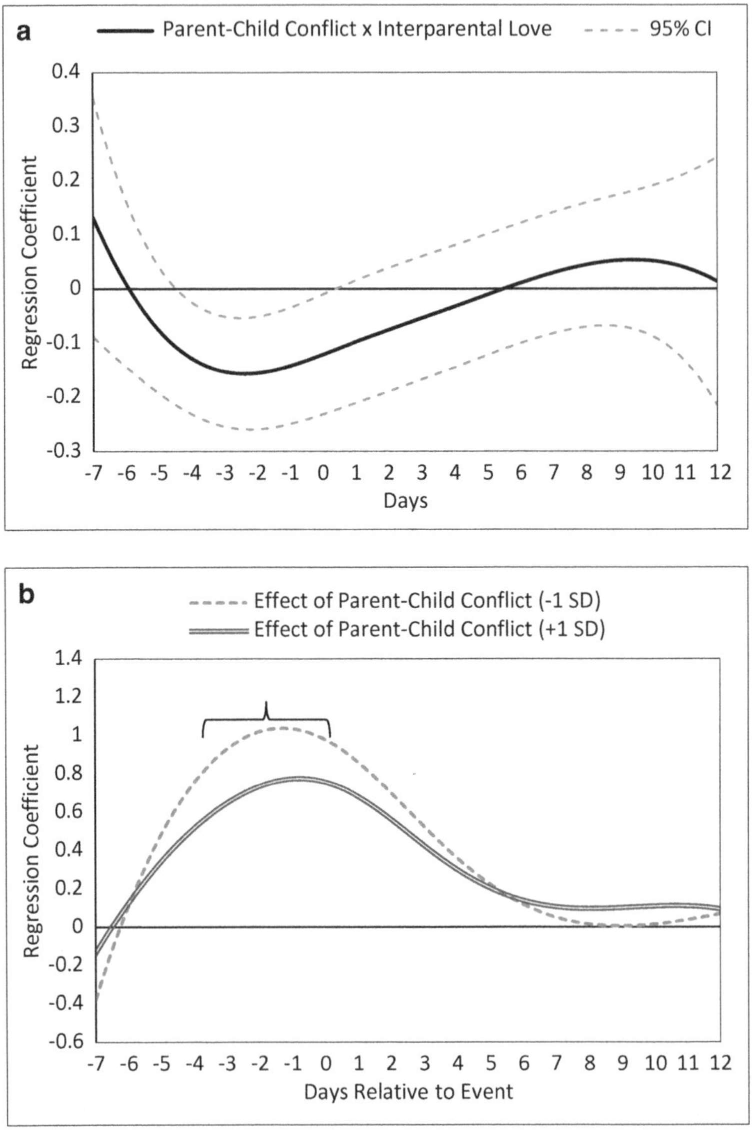

Fig. 6.8 (**a**) Effect of the interaction between parent-child conflict and interparental love on interparental conflict, across days relative to a conflict event (Day 0), controlling for conflict experienced on other days (with 95% confidence band). (**b**) Simple slopes for the association between parent-child conflict and interparental conflict across days, at higher (1 *SD* above mean level) and lower (1 *SD* below mean level) of interparental love, controlling for conflict experienced on other days. Brace indicates days on which significant differences in the association were observed between parents with higher versus lower levels of interparental love (i.e., days of significant moderation)

the association between levels of parent-child conflict and interparental conflict for several days leading up to the conflict event and on the day of the conflict event.

It should be noted that findings are based on self-reports, and, thus, social desirability may have impacted study findings. Also, we used self-reported data from only one parent's perspective; we do not have the perspective of the adolescent or the other parent. Further, associations modeled here should not be interpreted as causal, as potential confounders may explain the observed associations. Despite these limitations, these findings illustrate how TVEM can be used to estimate the dynamic nature of feelings and behaviors across a period of time and how covariates assessed at the day- and person-level may have nuanced time trends in their associations with outcomes. As noted earlier in this chapter, although MLM is a perfectly suitable approach to address certain questions using these data (e.g., whether an interparental conflict event was more common on days with higher reported parent-child conflict and whether this association differed depending on the level of interparental love), MLM generally does not take into account how these associations change across time, particularly when such change is nonlinear, as in this example. It is our hope that this empirical demonstration has shined a light on ways to think about time, and on new and exciting questions researchers can answer with their own ILD.

References

Braiker, H. B., & Kelley, H. H. (1979). Conflict in the development of close relationships. In R. L. Burgess & T. L. Huston (Eds.), *Social exchange in developing relationships* (pp. 135–168). Academic Press.

Fosco, G. M., & Lydon-Staley, D. M. (2019). A within-family examination of interparental conflict, cognitive appraisals, and adolescent mood and well-being. *Child Development, 90*(4), e421–e436.

Lanza, S. T., Vasilenko, S. A., Liu, X., Li, R., & Piper, M. E. (2014). Advancing the understanding of craving during smoking cessation attempts: A demonstration of the time-varying effect model. *Nicotine & Tobacco Research, 16*(Suppl_2), S127–S134.

Vasilenko, S. A., Piper, M. E., Lanza, S. T., Liu, X., Yang, J., & Li, R. (2014). Time-varying processes involved in smoking lapse in a randomized trial of smoking cessation therapies. *Nicotine & Tobacco Research, 16*(Suppl_2), S135–S143.

Chapter 7
Further Applications and Future Directions

Time-varying effect modeling (TVEM), also referred to as variable coefficient modeling in the statistical literature, is not a statistical innovation, per se, yet the impact of its application in the social, behavioral, and health sciences is far from realized. This is due in large part to researchers' lack of awareness of TVEM as a data analytic approach, the innovative research questions it can be used to address, and user-friendly software available for TVEM. Our hope is that this book introduces researchers to TVEM and that they add it to their analytic "toolbox." The research questions TVEM can be used to address complement those that can be addressed using techniques commonly used, including ANOVA, general linear modeling, logistic regression analysis, and growth curve modeling.

This final chapter is divided into three sections. First, we comment on several aspects of interpreting TVEM results that have come up many times in practice. Second, we discuss data and software considerations relevant to using TVEM. Third, we present a sample of topics that reflect ongoing and future work that will extend TVEM to even further advance research. These topics include alternative ways to conceptualize time and methodological innovations.

7.1 Comments on Interpreting TVEM Results

7.1.1 Inferring Causation

It is crucial that analysts remember that TVEM is a direct extension of linear regression, where the coefficients are estimated as a flexible, nonparametric function of time. At any particular moment in time, the coefficients are interpreted in the same way as in linear regression. That is, at any particular time, one unit higher on an independent variable is associated with a certain difference in the expected value of the dependent variable (which may or may not be statistically significant at that time

S. T. Lanza, A. N. Linden-Carmichael, *Time-Varying Effect Modeling for the Behavioral, Social, and Health Sciences*,
https://doi.org/10.1007/978-3-030-70944-0_7

point). When using TVEM with observational data, associations between independent variables and a dependent variable should not be interpreted as causal effects. Of course, if the independent variable is treatment condition in a randomized controlled trial, then inferring causality may be plausible. We encourage the reader to consider including covariates when analyzing data from observational studies, just as one would when fitting traditional linear regression, to facilitate interpretation of the association between an independent variable with an outcome while controlling for (or holding constant) other covariates in the model.

Including covariates in TVEM is straightforward in terms of model specification, but it can be important to consider whether covariates should be specified to have time-varying or time-invariant effects. Either type of effect is statistically appropriate, but there may be subtle differences in the interpretation of results. In reality, we rarely interpret regression coefficients in the presence of covariates with the level of specificity that would convey whether the effects of covariates were estimated as time-varying. We encourage researchers to be thoughtful about the desired interpretations of a coefficient function when additional covariates are included in the model. One pragmatic strategy for making this decision is to specify a model in which covariates have time-varying effects and a second model in which their effects are constant across time. If the coefficients for covariates do not show any variation across time then specifying them as having time-invariant effects in the final model is appropriate. If however they have effects that vary to some extent over time and the coefficient functions of interest show any change between the two models, careful thought should be given to the final model selection and its interpretation.

Propensity score modeling is a very useful tool for drawing more plausible causal inference when analyzing observational data (D'Agostino Jr, 1998; Lanza, Moore, & Butera, 2013; VanderWeele, 2006). In short, propensity scores are estimated for each individual such that, when a final analysis model is weighted by the inverse propensity scores, the coefficient of interest can be interpreted as if observations at different levels on the covariate are balanced across many observed characteristics. Although a thorough discussion of propensity score analysis for estimating causal effects is beyond the scope of this book, we believe future methodological work on integrating propensity score weighting in TVEM holds potential.

7.1.2 Lagged Associations and Mediation Analysis

Related to the issue of inferring causality, when using TVEM an analyst may need to consider potential time lags between independent variables and the dependent variable. Certainly, to plausibly infer causal effects, temporal ordering is necessary such that the independent variable occurs before (i.e., is measured prior to) the outcome. However, even when drawing causal inference is not a goal, it is important in any TVEM using longitudinal data or intensive longitudinal data (ILD) to consider whether to lag variables.

With TVEM, it is crucial to remember that associations are to be estimated as a function of time. That is, a regression coefficient at time t means that we expect a one-unit difference on a covariate to be associated with a difference in the outcome *at time t*. In a sense, this interpretation is agnostic to what the model says about times prior to or after t; our interpretation should always be grounded in drawing conclusions as a function of time. Let us consider a hypothetical daily diary study that assesses individuals each evening for 21 days, in which all participants began a new meditation program on Day 1. If we estimate the time-varying association between an indicator of whether the participants engaged in meditation practice that day and daily positive affect using concurrent (i.e., non-lagged) variables, our interpretation is clear: on Day t, engaging in meditation practice is associated with a particular expected difference in positive affect on that day; the estimated association may change across the 21-day period. This analysis would rely on data containing 21 pairs of concurrently measured variables for each individual. If however we wished to test the strength of association between daily meditation practice and next-day positive affect, we would lag the variables in the dataset such that meditation practice on Day t is the independent variable and positive affect on Day $t + 1$ is the dependent variable. The dataset becomes slightly smaller because, for each individual, there are only 20 pairs of lagged variables. More importantly, the interpretation of the association is as follows: engaging in meditation practice on Day t is associated with a particular expected difference in positive affect on Day $t + 1$; the estimated association may change across the 20-day period (i.e., predicting positive affect on study Days 2 through 21).

As with any longitudinal analysis, for lagged analyses to have interpretable results, the time that elapses between lags should be roughly the same across individuals. Further, when estimating a coefficient function in TVEM using lagged measures, it is important that the time that elapses between lags be roughly constant across the time axis. In the case of daily diary studies, the uniformity of spacing between measurements across participants and across the study period lends itself well to lagged analyses. However, when modeling more intensive ecological momentary assessments (EMA) using TVEM, careful thought should be given to the differences in time between assessments. Indeed, many EMA studies are designed to randomly sample across real-time thus by design, the lags between any two assessments may vary considerably.

Many social scientists focused on mechanisms of change over time have theories that lend themselves to mediation analysis. In its simplest terms, mediation models posit that an independent variable, X, causes a mediator variable, M, which in turn causes an outcome, Y (Mackinnon, 2008). This type of analysis has great conceptual appeal to test many theories, yet it requires that careful thought is given to issues of time lag and causal inference. We encourage researchers to consider specifically how they envision a mediational process would unfold across continuous time when assessments are made at discrete points in time. Further, currently, we are not aware of work to estimate time-varying indirect effects using TVEM; this is an important area for future methodological work.

7.1.3 How Do Multilevel Modeling, Growth Curve Modeling, and TVEM Differ?

A common misperception that researchers often have about TVEM when they first see plotted results is that the coefficient functions represent mean individual growth curves. For those of us who have become accustomed to estimating and interpreting growth curves using longitudinal data, this is a natural reaction to TVEM results. However, *results from growth curve modeling and TVEM have unilaterally different interpretations; the two modeling frameworks address inherently different research questions.* Below, we clarify the different goals of analyzing repeated-measures data (i.e., longitudinal data or ILD) using (1) multilevel modeling (MLM), also known as random effects modeling, (2) growth curve modeling, which is a special case of MLM, and (3) TVEM.

In general, MLM is used to estimate associations between variables in data that are characterized by some sort of clustering, or statistical nesting. Clustered data arise when individuals are nested within some type of structural unit (e.g., children nested in classrooms; adults nested within organizations) or when repeated measures are collected (i.e., repeated measures are nested within individuals). Using MLM to estimate an association between an independent variable (e.g., negative affect) and a dependent variable (e.g., nicotine craving) in repeated-measures data adjusts standard errors to account for the clustering of repeated observations within individuals. This approach also partitions the variance in an outcome into between-person variance (Level-2 variance, reflecting the degree to which people differ from each other on the outcome, craving) and within-person variance (Level-1 variance, reflecting the degree to which people differ from themselves on the outcome, craving, over time). MLM further allows researchers to model the effects of covariates at both levels; for example, individuals' typical negative affect can be included as a person-level covariate at Level 2, and individuals' deviations from their own mean negative affect can be included as a time-varying covariate at Level 1. This would allow one to address questions such as *"Across all days, what is the association between individuals' mean negative affect and the expected level of craving?"* and *"On days when individuals report negative affect one standard deviation higher than their mean, what is the expected difference in craving?"* Typically, MLM as described here is not used to model change across time or to consider whether coefficients vary across time; the association between negative affect and nicotine craving typically would be assumed to be a constant effect across the entire time interval.

One frequently used special case of MLM to analyze repeated-measures data is linear growth curve modeling. This approach is commonly used to estimate mean linear (or sometimes quadratic) growth curves in the outcome over time. Covariates of initial status (i.e., intercept, or estimated level on the outcome at time 0) and slope (i.e., linear rate of change over time in the outcome) can be included; however, this approach typically does *not* allow associations between variables to vary with time. For example, in a smoking cessation trial in which individuals are assessed repeatedly after a quit attempt, a growth curve analysis typically would be used to address questions such as *"What is the mean linear growth curve that reflects individuals' craving over the course of the study?"* and *"What is the association between initial (Day 1) negative affect and initial craving, and between initial negative affect and individuals' linear rate of change in craving?"* Importantly, a figure showing the mean growth curve for craving over time does reflect the average linear curve. Conceptually, this is analogous to estimating linear change over time in craving for each individual and averaging across those lines to convey the average growth curve or trajectory in craving across the study period.

The interpretation of figures showing TVEM results can be in subtle—or stark—contrast to the interpretation of a growth curve. First, consider an intercept-only time-varying effect model of craving over time. This curve may be nonlinear (or even quite complex across time), and reflects the estimated mean craving *across individuals at each particular time t*. In other words, it is a sophisticated approach to estimating mean craving as a function of time that is conceptually analogous to simply plotting the sample mean craving at each time point and smoothing across the points. Now consider including negative affect as a time-varying covariate, specified so that its effect may vary nonparametrically across time. This TVEM specification enables population-level questions to be addressed, including *"What is the expected level of craving across the course of the study, and what is the shape of change over time?"* and *"What is the association between negative affect and craving at each point across time in the study, and at which times is that association statistically significant?"* Just as traditional linear regression coefficients (and correlation coefficients, more simply) reflect the estimated population-level association between an independent variable and a dependent variable, so does each point across time shown in a coefficient function for the association in TVEM. TVEM allows researchers to explore the possibility that—in addition to time-varying covariates changing over time (e.g., negative affect in the previous example)—associations do in fact change as flexible functions of time, and the shape of change over time may be highly complex. In a special issue of *Nicotine and Tobacco Research* on EMA to study nicotine use, Lanza, Vasilenko, Liu, Li, and Piper (2014) provide a demonstration of using TVEM to estimate the time-varying association between negative affect and craving as a function of time since smoking quit attempt. A study by Vasilenko et al. (2014) appearing in the same special issue examined data from the same smoking study and provides a direct comparison between MLM and TVEM to analyze ILD.

7.2 Extensions of TVEM and Future Directions

7.2.1 Moving Beyond Time: Other Applications of TVEM

In addition to thinking of time as real-time (i.e., *calendar or clock time*), researchers can think of time more creatively to address a broad set of questions. For example, Lanza, Vasilenko, and Russell (2016) published a manuscript in *Psychology of*

Addictive Behaviors that demonstrated four different metrics of time that can be conceptualized in TVEM and applied to cross-sectional or longitudinal data. Three of these metrics were demonstrated in this book: *developmental time* to examine age-varying associations between heavy alcohol use and cannabis use, similar to what is presented in Chap. 4 of this book; *historical time* to understand how the association between cannabis use attitudes and cannabis use behavior has changed between 1976 and 2013, similar to what is presented in Chap. 5 of this book; and changes in cannabis use as a function of *time relative to an event*, in this case the birth of first child, similar to what is presented in Chap. 6 of this book.

One additional metric of time was demonstrated in this manuscript: *age of onset*. Age of onset of cannabis use was examined in relation to the prevalence of adult cannabis use to identify ages of first use that are particularly risky. Lanza et al. (2016) analyzed data from a large, national, cross-sectional study. Figure 7.1 (which reproduces Fig. 5 from the published manuscript) was created by specifying a time-varying effect model using just three variables from the dataset: a continuous variable indicating age of first use of cannabis (ranging from 10 to 40 years, specified as the time variable), a binary indicator of past-year cannabis use in adulthood, and a binary indicator of sex. Based on an intercept-only TVEM, Fig. 7.1a shows that the overall rate of adult cannabis use was highest among those who initiated use around ages 10–11, with decreasing risk through the onset of about age 18. Sex differences in this study show that age of onset plays a somewhat stronger role among male individuals, particularly for those who initiated use at age 10 (Fig. 7.1b). Among female individuals, ages of onset around ages 10–13 conferred similar risk for adult use. A similar study was conducted to examine the age of onset of first nicotine use as a risk factor for adult nicotine dependence (Lanza & Vasilenko, 2015). Peak risk was associated with onset at age 11, with an elevated risk through about age 20; sex differences revealed heightened sensitivity among female individuals compared to male individuals through age 21.

In addition to these more obvious ways to conceive of time, the TVEM software can be a convenient way to examine an incredibly broad set of questions about nonlinear associations. That is, a continuous variable that has nothing to do with time could be specified for the x-axis. Several substance use studies demonstrate this approach using what are essentially *exposure variables on the x-axis instead of time*, for example, specifying the number of days in the past month one used cannabis (Dierker, Selya, Lanza, Li, & Rose, 2018) or number of alcoholic drinks (Linden-Carmichael, Russell, & Lanza, 2019) in place of the "time" variable. For example, in Linden-Carmichael, Russell, and Lanza (2019), the prevalence of young adults meeting criteria for a past-year alcohol use disorder (AUD) was modeled as a function of number of drinks consumed during a typical drinking occasion during the past year. This model demonstrated how one's risk of experiencing an AUD increased as a flexible function of each additional drink reported during a typical occasion. As shown in Fig. 7.2, the rate of AUD increased for male (black line) and female (gray line) young adults steeply until approximately 10–12 drinks after which the risk for AUD plateaued. Significant sex differences at specific numbers of typical drinks are denoted with boxes.

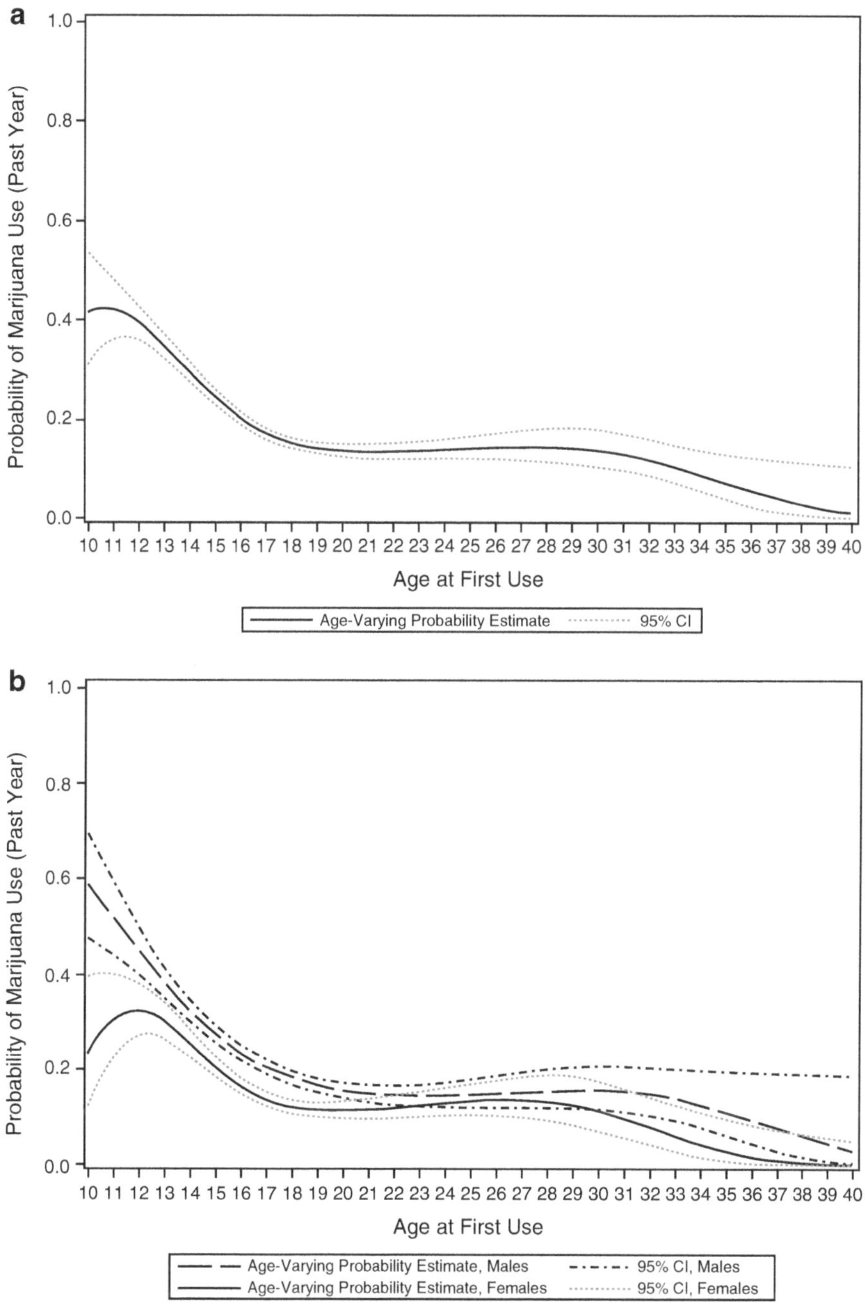

Fig. 7.1 Estimated probability of adult marijuana use as a function of age of onset (a) overall and (b) by gender. Reproduced with permission from Lanza, S. T., Vasilenko, S. A., & Russell, M. A. (2016). Time-varying effect modeling to address new questions in behavioral research: Examples in marijuana use. Psychology of Addictive Behaviors, 30(8), 939-954. American Psychological Association

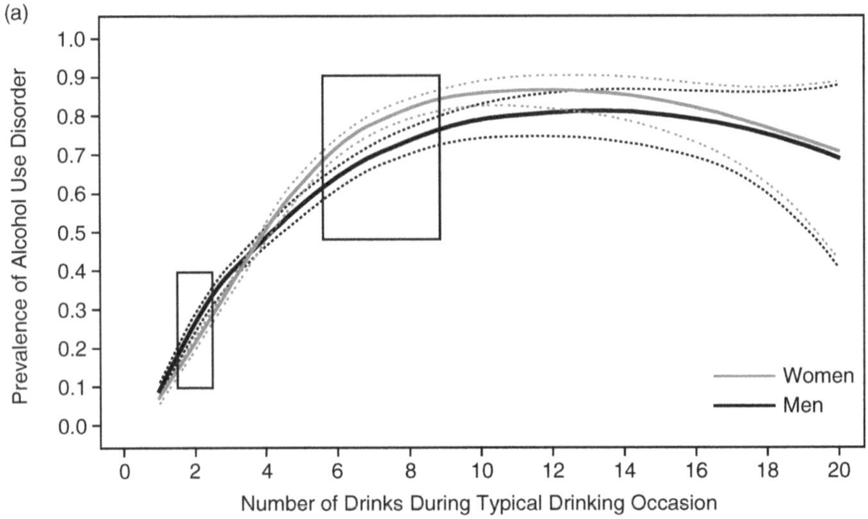

Fig. 7.2 Estimated prevalence of alcohol use disorder as a function of the number of drinks typically consumed on a drinking occasion in the past year, separately for men and women. Boxes indicate number of drinks at which gender differences in the prevalence of alcohol use disorder were significant. Reproduced with permission from Linden-Carmichael, A. N., Russell, M. A., and Lanza, S. T. (2019). Flexibly modeling alcohol use disorder risk: How many drinks should we count? Psychology of Addictive Behaviors, 33(1), 50-57. American Psychological Association

7.2.2 TVEM for Zero-Inflated Count Outcomes

Count data on health behaviors or related outcomes often contain more zeroes than would be expected in a true Poisson distribution. In regression analysis, this is often addressed by using options such as hurdle models, zero-inflated Poisson models, negative binomial models, or zero-inflated negative binomial models. A preliminary SAS macro for fitting TVEM with zero-inflated Poisson data has been developed (Li, Tan, Huang, Wagner, & Yang, 2015). However, it does not have all features that are available in the TVEM macros for continuous or binary outcomes. Additionally, it is not recommended for general use with longitudinal data because it does not take into account within-subject correlation.

The computational complexity in taking longitudinal correlation into account in a Poisson TVEM arises from the fact that zero-inflated models treat the sample as a mixture of two classes. For example, when modeling an outcome such as number of alcoholic drinks in the past week, a zero-inflated Poisson model posits that there are two classes of individuals: nonusers, who never report having any drinks (i.e., always have a 0 on the outcome by definition) and users, who typically report a nonzero value but could potentially report 0 drinks for a particular time period. Class membership might be treated as a permanent (but latent) characteristic of an individual, or might be allowed to vary over time. Allowing both the class membership and the amount of use given membership in the user class to vary over time and allowing the two parts of the model to be correlated over time in a realistic way were challenging to implement in SAS. The current SAS %TVEM macro for count data is valid for cross-sectional data; however, it is possible that future research might provide guidance for fitting these models in a different way, perhaps using a Bayesian approach that is more flexible.

7.2.3 Software, Missing Data, and Sample Size Considerations

Statistical software development for a variety of complex models is advancing rapidly. At the time of this writing, the SAS %TVEM macros developed by our team represent the most well-established, user-friendly, and well-documented software to fit TVEM; thus, we demonstrate all models in this book using SAS (https://prevention.psu.edu/books/tvem/). Work by colleagues has begun for developing software to fit time-varying effect models in R, which would provide a free and open-source alternative to using SAS.[1] Related statistical models may be estimated in Mplus (Muthén & Muthén, 1998-2017) under the framework of dynamic structural equation modeling (Asparouhov, Hamaker, & Muthén, 2018).

Missing data is an issue that essentially every applied researcher must consider. TVEM uses all available data, with observations excluded if there is missing data on either a covariate or the outcome. In short, current software uses listwise deletion at the level of an assessment; for example, in an ILD study if an individual provides data on 30 out of a possible 40 assessments, that individual still contributes 30 assessments in the analysis. When analyzing cross-sectional data however if an individual has missing data on one of the analysis variables they are eliminated from the analysis. Missing data results in a loss of efficiency in parameter estimation. The larger concern, of course, is if participants at different times (e.g., ages) are more or less likely to provide data, thereby biasing TVEM results. For example, if younger adults who have contracted a sexually transmitted infection (STI) are less likely to respond to a question about this topic compared to older adults, the rate of STIs may appear to be lower than it truly is in young adulthood.

Multiple imputation (Schafer, 1997) may be a useful solution to address missing data in the case of cross-sectional data and, in some cases, longitudinal data. In this approach, the data would be imputed under an inclusive, most likely multivariate normal model, although it is unclear if or how the values of the spline basis functions would need to be included in the imputation model. The same TVEM specification would be applied to each (say, 20) imputed dataset. The challenge would be for the analyst to combine coefficient functions—and the corresponding standard errors—across imputations to derive the final estimates. We see this as a potentially fruitful solution to missing data that merits further study.

---

[1] Interested readers can find an experimental testing version, which does not include all of the features in the SAS macros, at https://github.com/dziakj1/TvemPackage

Longitudinal studies face an important source of missingness, attrition, which refers to study drop-out among individuals who participated in the first wave of data collection. Some longitudinal panel studies, particularly those that employ survey weights to help generalize findings to the larger population, provide special "longitudinal weights" at each wave that are designed to make the sample still participating at that wave (i.e., those who have not dropped out of the study) more generalizable to the population. We recommend using longitudinal weights when available for TVEM applied to panel data. For example, the first four waves of data collected in the National Longitudinal Survey of Adolescent to Adult Health (Add Health; (Harris, 2013)) span adolescence and young adulthood. By applying Wave 4 longitudinal weights in TVEM, all assessments from individuals who dropped out of the study prior to Wave 4 are excluded from the analysis. The weights are applied to make the smaller sample still present at Wave 4 representative and to ensure that the composition of the sample is the same across all waves. As an example, the empirical study by Mak, Fosco, and Lanza (2020) applied longitudinal weights when using TVEM to analyze data from the Add Health study.

In the case of ILD, the issue of missing data often is a complex one regardless of the method of analysis being used. Often, EMA are obtained at random times throughout the day (within constraints, e.g., one prompt during every 2-hr window). If, by design, such assessments are meant to sample real-time, then the implications of missing data must be considered carefully. For example, if individuals are assessed randomly across time during a study, at what exact times would one choose to impute data? In general, missing data in ILD studies is an important area for future research regardless of the analytic approach being used to analyze the data.

Sample size requirements for TVEM are not yet well understood. In particular, further research is needed on how to consider statistical power to detect complex curve shapes. However, recall that TVEM is a direct extension of multiple linear regression such that regression coefficients are estimated as a function of continuous time. Because statistical inference based on the linear regression model is made at specific time points, it may be useful to consider statistical power at a particular time or times using well-developed power formulae for regression analysis. For example, one could determine the sample size needed to detect a particular linear association between a covariate and an outcome with power of 0.80 or greater; this would provide strong guidance as to whether statistical power is likely to be adequate to test this association across different points of time. One reassuring note is that, because we are relying on pointwise confidence bands that facilitate hypothesis testing at a particular time point, confidence intervals around the coefficient function will be wider at times when data are more sparse. Thus, researchers can be assured that the confidence with which we interpret and make inference about time-varying effects will reflect the amount of information we have to support our findings at each time. Finally, several examples in this book are based on large datasets; in these cases, the researcher need not be concerned about whether the sample size is sufficient to use TVEM. Rather, the concern is that even relatively small effects may be statistically significant. As with any statistical analysis, the clinical/practical implications of a finding should be taken into account along with its statistical significance.

7.2.4 Random Effects for Spline Coefficients

The %TVEM macro with B-splines does optionally allow random effects in the form of subject-specific additive intercept constants (i.e., random intercepts) and subject-specific linear slopes (i.e., random slopes). However, these intercepts and slopes are still added on to the time-varying coefficients. The spline coefficients themselves are not treated as random effects but are assumed to be the same for every participant. Coefficients are not allowed to vary nonlinearly with time while also being different for every subject; this would be too complex to fit, resulting in problems with identification and computation of the estimates. If Bayesian priors were used for each coefficient and each knot, it would be possible to fit a subject-specific time-varying effect model with random coefficients, by using the prior information to keep the shapes of the estimated functions similar while not being identical. However, this approach would be computationally challenging. We believe that interpretation of such a model however where spline coefficients could vary across individuals, may pose some challenges in terms of interpretation and generalizability of findings. Grimm, Ram, and Hamagami (2011) describe options for including random effects in nonlinear parametric models, although spline-based modeling is not the focus of their paper.

7.2.5 MixTVEM: Latent Classes of Individuals Defined by TVEM Coefficients

Besides random effects, another possible approach to including heterogeneity between subjects in a time-varying effect model, particularly when analyzing ILD, would be to incorporate latent classes (part of the finite mixture modeling framework; see McLachlan and Peel (2000)). In finite mixture models, it is assumed that the population of interest consists of different types of people, with members of the same (unobserved) latent class being more similar to each other than to members of other classes. It is not assumed that class membership is known or observed. The word "finite" means that it is assumed that there are only a small number of such classes, rather than every person having their own unique model. Random effects models can be thought of as a kind of infinite mixture (Lindsay, 1995). The MixTVEM approach proposed by Dziak, Li, Tan, Shiffman, and Shiyko (2015) combines finite mixture modeling with TVEM, specifically by estimating a separate time-varying effect model, resulting in differently shaped coefficient functions, within each latent class. For example, the mean of the outcome Y_i for class c at time t might be modeled as $\beta_{0c}(t) + \beta_{1c}(t)X_i$, meaning that the relationship between X_i and Y_i depends both on time and on latent class. Dziak et al. (2015) studied self-reported urge to smoke nicotine, as predicted by negative affect, in a sample of adults who were trying to quit smoking and provided intensive data across several weeks. They identified three latent classes: a mild class that had generally low and decreasing self-rated urge; a severe class that had high self-rated urge that did not decrease much over time and that was related to momentary negative affect; and a moderate class that had highly variable self-rated urge which was also related to momentary negative affect, although less so over time.

Many choices must be made in fitting a MixTVEM, and further research is needed to better guide researchers in making them. For example, a covariate can be specified as a predictor of the time-varying outcome as in standard TVEM, where the coefficient function can vary across latent classes. Alternatively, that same covariate can be used to predict latent class membership. However, for interpretability and model identification it would be difficult to use the same covariate for both. Additionally, best practices to select the optimal number of latent classes in MixTVEM requires further methodological research. Syntax to fit the MixTVEM in R or SAS, for the case of a normal outcome, is available at https://github.com/dziakj1/MixTVEM, although this syntax is not as user-friendly or extensively documented as the TVEM macro in SAS. This syntax also does not accommodate sample weights. The computational and statistical performance of MixTVEM was studied in a recent technical paper by Yang, Shao, and Cai (2019).

7.2.6 Time-Varying Coefficients in Latent Class Analysis

An alternative way to combine mixture modeling with TVEM, informally known as LCA-TVEM, was proposed in Linden-Carmichael, Dziak, and Lanza (2019) and Bray, Dziak, and Lanza (2019). Essentially LCA-TVEM refers to TVEM where the outcome is a latent class variable. The latent class parameters (i.e., class membership probabilities and item-response probabilities linking covariates with class membership) are modeled as functions of time, either using polynomials or splines. The latent classes themselves are measured using several observed indicators as in classic latent class analysis (see, e.g., Collins & Lanza, 2010; Lanza, Collins, Lemmon, & Schafer, 2007). In LCA-TVEM, a single TVEM applies to every participant, but latent class membership (measured by a set of indicator variables) is itself the outcome. However, as with MixTVEM, LCA-TVEM is currently computationally challenging.

The simplest form of LCA-TVEM is to conduct a latent class analysis and include a covariate reflecting time (t) that is centered near the midpoint of time in the study, as well as covariates reflecting t^2, t^3, and so on, as covariates of class membership. Centering t in this way reduces multicollinearity of the polynomial terms. Time-varying class membership probabilities can be graphed, analogous to intercept-only TVEM. A substantive covariate and its product with the polynomial indicators of time also can be included as covariates to examine time-varying associations of that covariate with latent class membership. To date, LCA-TVEM has only been used to analyze cross-sectional data, in which different people have different values of time (e.g., age) and may have sample weights, but measurements are only taken on a given individual once. This avoids needing to allow individuals to change latent class membership across time, which could make the model

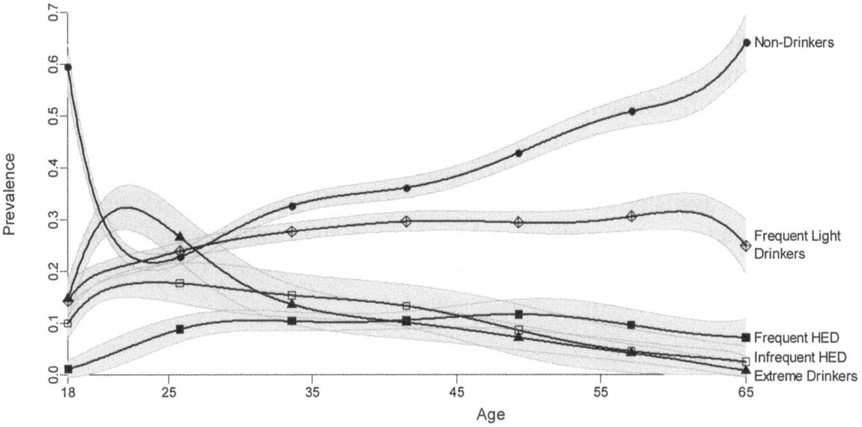

Fig. 7.3 Prevalence of five latent classes defined by past-year alcohol use behaviors as a function of age. Reprinted from Bray, B. C., Dziak, J. J., and Lanza, S. T. (2019). Age trends in alcohol use behavior patterns among US adults ages 18–65. Drug and Alcohol Dependence, 205, 107688, with permission from Elsevier

considerably more complicated in terms of computation and interpretation. However, at least in principle, it would be possible to link TVEM not only with latent class analysis but with latent transition analysis in which class membership is dynamic.

Several empirical studies demonstrate simple cases of LCA-TVEM, including Linden-Carmichael, Dziak, and Lanza (2019) and Bray et al. (2019). Bray and colleagues estimated alcohol use latent class membership of adults in a large, national, cross-sectional study. Class membership probabilities were estimated as a function of centered $t, t^2, \ldots, t^6$, allowing the prevalence of each latent class to vary quite flexibly across ages 18–65. Importantly, at any particular age, the proportion of individuals expected to be in each latent class sum to 1.0 thus their relative prevalence changes with time. The five classes were Non-Drinkers, Frequent Light Drinkers, Infrequent Heavy Episodic Drinkers, Frequent Heavy Episodic Drinkers, and Extreme Drinkers. As shown in Fig. 7.3 (which reproduces Fig. 1 from the published manuscript), Non-Drinkers were most prevalent across all ages except during the early 20s, when Extreme Drinkers were more prevalent. Prevalences of the Infrequent Heavy Episodic Drinkers and Extreme Drinkers classes peaked around ages 22–24, but the prevalence of the Frequent Heavy Episodic Drinkers class peaked around age 49.

7.3 Conclusion

Our primary goal in writing this book was to introduce researchers to TVEM so that they can gain new insight into processes that unfold across time. Over time, we anticipate that additional methodological advancements to this method will be made to further expand the set of research questions that can be addressed with TVEM. In addition to the text presented in this book, excellent online resources on this analytic method can be found at the companion website for this book (https://prevention.psu.edu/books/tvem/). These resources include annotated syntax for all models specified in the empirical examples presented in this volume, a list of recommended readings, answers to frequently asked questions, and additional learning materials. We also make available a set of materials designed for instructors, specifically those who teach graduate-level methods, who wish to include a module on TVEM in their course. We look forward to reading about many new studies by researchers who apply TVEM in their work.

References

Asparouhov, T., Hamaker, E. L., & Muthén, B. (2018). Dynamic structural equation models. *Structural Equation Modeling, 25*(3), 359–388.

Bray, B. C., Dziak, J. J., & Lanza, S. T. (2019). Age trends in alcohol use behavior patterns among US adults ages 18–65. *Drug and Alcohol Dependence, 205*, 107689.

Collins, L. M., & Lanza, S. T. (2010). *Latent class and latent transition analysis: With applications in the social, behavioral, and health sciences*. John Wiley & Sons.

D'Agostino, R. B., Jr. (1998). Propensity score methods for bias reduction in the comparison of a treatment to a non-randomized control group. *Statistics in Medicine, 17*(19), 2265–2281.

Dierker, L., Selya, A., Lanza, S., Li, R., & Rose, J. (2018). Depression and marijuana use disorder symptoms among current marijuana users. *Addictive Behaviors, 76*, 161–168.

Dziak, J. J., Li, R., Tan, X., Shiffman, S., & Shiyko, M. P. (2015). Modeling intensive longitudinal data with mixtures of nonparametric trajectories and time-varying effects. *Psychological Methods, 20*(4), 444–469.

Grimm, K. J., Ram, N., & Hamagami, F. (2011). Nonlinear growth curves in developmental research. *Child Development, 82*(5), 1357–1371.

Harris, K. M. (2013). *The Add Health study: Design and accomplishments*. Carolina Population Center, University of North Carolina at Chapel Hill.

Lanza, S. T., Collins, L. M., Lemmon, D. R., & Schafer, J. L. (2007). PROC LCA: A SAS procedure for latent class analysis. *Structural Equation Modeling, 14*(4), 671–694.

Lanza, S. T., Moore, J. E., & Butera, N. M. (2013). Drawing causal inferences using propensity scores: A practical guide for community psychologists. *American Journal of Community Psychology, 52*(3-4), 380–392.

Lanza, S. T., & Vasilenko, S. A. (2015). New methods shed light on age of onset as a risk factor for nicotine dependence. *Addictive Behaviors, 50*, 161–164.

Lanza, S. T., Vasilenko, S. A., Liu, X., Li, R., & Piper, M. E. (2014). Advancing the understanding of craving during smoking cessation attempts: A demonstration of the time-varying effect model. *Nicotine & Tobacco Research, 16*(Suppl_2), S127–S134.

Lanza, S. T., Vasilenko, S. A., & Russell, M. A. (2016). Time-varying effect modeling to address new questions in behavioral research: Examples in marijuana use. *Psychology of Addictive Behaviors, 30*(8), 939–954.

Li, R., Tan, X., Huang, L., Wagner, A. T., & Yang, J. (2015). *%TVEM_zip (time-varying effect model) SAS macro users' guide*. The Methodology Center, Penn State.

Linden-Carmichael, A. N., Russell, M. A., & Lanza, S. T. (2019). Flexibly modeling alcohol use disorder risk: How many drinks should we count? *Psychology of Addictive Behaviors, 33*(1), 50--57.

Linden-Carmichael, A. N., Russell, M. A., & Lanza, S. T. (2019). Flexibly modeling alcohol use disorder risk: How many drinks should we count? *Psychology of Addictive Behaviors, 33*(1), 50.

Lindsay, B. G. (1995). Mixture models: Theory, geometry and applications (monograph). In *NSF-CBMS Regional Conference Series in Probability and Statistics, Volume 5* (pp. i-163). JSTOR.

MacKinnon, D. (2008). *Introduction to statistical mediation analysis*. Taylor & Francis Group LLC.

Mak, H. W., Fosco, G. M., & Lanza, S. T. (2020). Dynamic associations of parent-adolescent closeness and friend support with adolescent depressive symptoms across ages 12–19. *Journal of Research on Adolescence*. Advance online publication. 10.1111/jora.12597.

McLachlan, G., & Peel, D. (2000). *Finite mixture models*. Wiley.

Muthén, L. K., & Muthén, B. O. (1998-2017). *Mplus user's guide, eighth edition*. Muthén & Muthén.

Schafer, J. L. (1997). *Analysis of incomplete multivariate data*. Chapman and Hall/CRC.

VanderWeele, T. (2006). The use of propensity score methods in psychiatric research. *International Journal of Methods in Psychiatric Research, 15*(2), 95–103.

Vasilenko, S. A., Piper, M. E., Lanza, S. T., Liu, X., Yang, J., & Li, R. (2014). Time-varying processes involved in smoking lapse in a randomized trial of smoking cessation therapies. *Nicotine & Tobacco Research, 16*(Suppl_2), S135–S143.

Yang, J., Shao, M., & Cai, G. (2019). On the performance of MixTVEM: A simulation study. *Communications in Statistics-Simulation and Computation, 48*(9), 2830–2844.

Index

S. T. Lanza, A. N. Linden-Carmichael, *Time-Varying Effect Modeling for the Behavioral, Social, and Health Sciences*,
https://doi.org/10.1007/978-3-030-70944-0

The manufacturer's authorised representative in the EU is Springer Nature Customer Service Centre GmbH, Europaplatz 3, 69115 Heidelberg, Germany. If you have any concerns regarding our products, please contact ProductSafety@springernature.com

Printed and bound by CPI Group (UK) Ltd, Croydon, CR0 4YY
30/09/2026
02225608-0013